Periodontal Diseases
A Manual of Diagnosis, Treatment and Maintenance
Hans R Preus and Lars Laurell

Periodontal Diseases

A Manual of
Diagnosis, Treatment and Maintenance

by

Hans R Preus and Lars Laurell

Quintessence Publishing Co. Ltd.

London, Berlin, Chicago, Copenhagen, Paris, Milan, Barcelona,
Istanbul, São Paulo, Tokyo, New Dehli, Moscow, Prague, Warsaw

British Library Cataloguing in Publication Data

Preus, H. R.
  Periodontal diseases : a manual of diagnosis, treatment and maintenance
  1. Periodontal disease – Diagnosis 2. Periodontal disease – Treatment
  I. Title II. Laurell, L.
  617.6'32

ISBN 1850970726

ISBN 1-85097-072-6

Preface

An increasingly disturbing trend for dental clinicians is the tendency to refrain from diagnosing and properly treating periodontal diseases. The most common litigation brought against the profession today is initiated because dentists have not diagnosed and treated periodontal diseases properly. Studies by Lie and Mellingen from the University of Bergen, Norway, show that Norwegian dentists spend only 3.1 minutes per patient per year on treatment of periodontal diseases. Furthermore, they also reported that 90% of the patients that were enrolled at the Department of Periodontology, Dental Faculty, University of Bergen, did not know that they had the disease, and that they had never received any information on this topic from their dentists despite regular visits. The remaining 10% had received inadequate treatment and information.

This book is intended as an update in clinical periodontology and periodontics, where new and old principles for treatment are discussed and evaluated. We introduce several new concepts and ideas, which hopefully may contribute to you and your team's success rate in treating periodontal diseases. Our intention is to build upon the knowledge that dentists and hygienists have gained already from graduate training programs. We also aim to provide guidance in the modern diagnosis of patients with periodontitis, correct treatments, referral and follow-up routines, as well as methods for the retrospective evaluation of treatment. It has not been our intention to write a full textbook, but rather a manual for the interested clinician – a manual that takes a stand on different questions, describes treatment regimes and provides you, the reader, with readily accessible answers to most of your clinical questions on periodontics.

In conclusion, we hope this handbook will prove to be valuable in your clinical practice, allowing you to help more of your patients suffering from periodontitis, thereby becoming an even more successful dentist. Treating periodontal diseases is not easy, you need strategies – and this manual presents them to you.

The authors wish to thank Professor Harald Löe, the former Director of MIDR, USA, for his extensive help in editing the English edition of this book.

Contents

Chapter 4
THE USE OF ANTIBIOTICS IN PERIODONTAL DISEASE CONTROL   55

CHAPTER 1

Diagnosis of periodontal diseases

Different types of periodontal diseases

In their 20+-year **longitudinal** study "The natural history of periodontal disease" Drs Löe, Aanerud and Boysen described a population in Sri Lanka that never visited a dentist nor practiced any systematic form of oral hygiene. In a series of articles based on these studies the authors claimed that they were able to classify the progression of periodontal diseases in this population based on the rate of destruction into 3 categories: *Rapidly Progressing* (8%), *Moderately Progressing* (81%) and *Non Progressing* (11%). Their diagnostic parameter was *attachment loss per unit time*. In order to describe the seriousness of the disease Dr. Löe used the *rate of attachment loss*. These findings have later been acknowledged and extended by other researchers all around the world. Thus, this is what we find in most populations, and may use in our interpretation of diagnosis and treatment of this group of dieases

Cross-sectional studies have shown that more than 50% of all individuals over the age of 40 years suffer from some form of periodontal disease, and that 8–12% suffer from severe forms of the disease. From the age of 50, more than 25% of the population has advanced, destructive periodontal disease.

In other words, there are *several forms of periodontal diseases* primarily governed by the individual's susceptibility to infection – and there are few, but important, differences in

this picture from country to country. From our clinical practices we recognize the special periodontal disease that affects smokers, the stressed stockbroker or divorcee and the ones with poor oral hygiene. We should also include those patients who, through no fault of their own, experience continuing attachment loss, despite meticulous oral hygiene practices and repeated check-ups with scaling every 3–4 months. Professor Roy Page once described periodontal disease as: "a family of related diseases that differ in etiology, natural history disease progression and response to therapy, but have a common chain of events." In other words, most periodontal diseases look alike clinically, but are different in bacteriology, host response (immunology), and with respect to environmental factors – like oral hygiene, drug use/abuse, smoking and other. That is why we tend to separate the periodontal diseases into groups like: *Aggressive periodontitis* that often strikes children or young adults, and *Chronic Periodontitis*, which normally is diagnosed in adults and the elderly. Even if the prerequisite for the development of marginal periodontitis requires the presence of specific bacteria (i.e. *Actinobacillus actinomycetemcomitans, Porphyromonas gingivalis, Prevotella intermedia*, etc.) there are several known and probably unknown risk factors and markers, which increase the risk for development of periodontal diseases. Among those known are diabetes mellitus, some im-

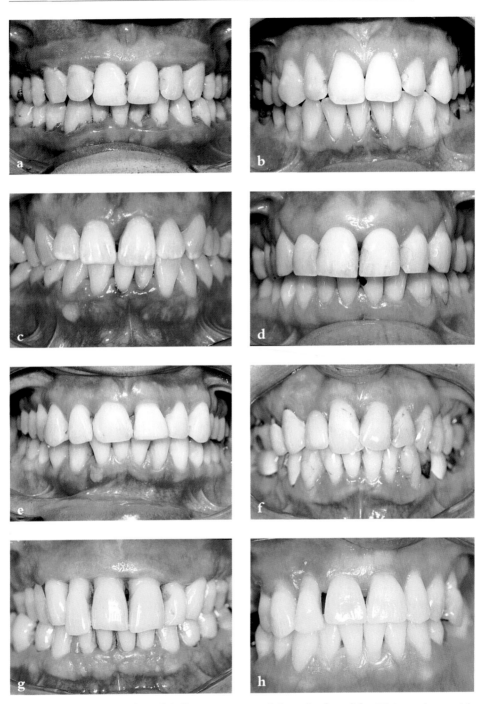

Fig 1 a – h **Every patient his/her own special periodontitis.** Eight patients with different forms of destructive periodontal diseases. a; man – 27 years, b; woman – 29 years, c; woman – 29 years, d; woman – 30 years, e; woman – 36 years, d; woman – 30 years, e; woman – 36 years, g; man – 31 years, h; woman – 47 years.

munological disorders and behaviors that enhance the possibility for infection onset and disease progression.

The fact that periodontal diseases are more or less different, and that they therefore must be subject to different treatment modalities, emphasizes the need for careful diagnosis. Clinicians must diagnose the different infections microbiologically as well as immunologically, and use the knowledge of how systemic responses and environmental factors influence the onset and the progression of the disease. As clinicians, we have tended to view periodontal diseases as one single disease, and treated every patient according to a standard, routine concept. This approach has undeniably had some success, because the type of periodontitis often haphazardly fitted this standard treatment modality. However, all too often this conventional treatment failed, and led to discouragement among the clinicians and the notion that these diseases are more or less untreatable.

In this book we suggest that routine, conventional treatment is effective only in cases where the periodontal infection has an uncomplicated etiology and pathogenesis, and where the treatment for one reason or another stops the destructive process. On the other hand, if we accept the concept that all periodontal diseases are different, but only look alike, we also embrace the idea that several treatment modalities are needed in order to provide adequate treatment for our patients. It is therefore essential that the dental team must individualize the understanding of the patient, the disease and the treatment in order to achieve *predictable* positive results.

The prerequisite for success is the realization that: "every patient has his/her own special periodontitis." (Fig. 1)

The slowly progressive periodontal diseases are the diseases most commonly encountered in clinical practice. Treating these infections is not too time or resource consuming. The slowly progressive peri-

odontal diseases occur – or are discovered – in the 30–40 year-old patient group, are mostly associated with the presence of subgingival dental plaque and calculus, and caused by 'non-specific' infections. The infections start as a result of accumulation of subgingival bacterial plaque, and it is these bacterial accumulations and their toxic products that elicit the inflammatory responses of the tissue. In other words, it is the cumulative effect of all (or most of) the plaque bacteria that causes the disease.

The rapidly progressive periodontal diseases are not the ones most commonly encountered in general dental practice. Dr. Löe and his collaborators found that 8% of all 40-year-olds in his study suffered from such rapidly progressing diseases. Studies from other countries, like Sweden, report that the prevalence of rapidly progressing diseases varies from 8–12%, and similar proportions have been reported for the USA and the UK.

The rapidly progressive disease is normally localized in single teeth or sites, but may also be more or less generalized, and show aggressive progression despite adequate oral hygiene and self care. These forms of the disease are regarded as specific infections.

In the medical literature, a specific infection is defined as a condition, in which one bacterial type causes one disease. In periodontology this does not apply. The subgingival dental plaque (biofilm) contains several hundred different microorganisms and an unknown number of fungi as well as human and bacterial viruses (bacteriophages). Thus we have made a definition that is more related to ecological microbiology, suggesting that a specific periodontal infection is an infection where certain microbial ecosystems are related to disease, while other are compatible with periodontal health. Some researchers have opined that all oral bacteria present in the periodontal pocket may produce disease, given optimal conditions, and that some bacteria (or ecosystems) may produce disease more consistently than others, simply, because they are better adapted or more virulent. These characteristics may also explain their survival during passage (transmission) from one person to the other, especially within families.

Several types of periodontitis in the same mouth (Fig. 2)

Rapidly and moderately progressing periodontitis may occur alone, or concomitantly in the same dentition. It is of the essence to separate the two – especially in those cases where several types of periodontitis occur side by side. In addition, it is common to find gingivitis in varying degree in areas with destructive periodontal disease, as well as in areas where no loss of attachment is clinically evident. Thus, it is important to have several diagnostic tools at hand, and to observe the lesions over time, in order to detect and distinguish such combinations of infections in one and the same mouth.

Gingivitis

Gingivitis is located in the gingiva. It is caused by non-specific infections and occurs as a result of supra- and subgingival accumulations of bacterial plaque. Chronic gingivitis is a reversible lesion. The clinical symptoms are: edema, increased tissue temperature, occasional tenderness, redness and provoked or unprovoked bleeding. The removal of subgingival plaque results in a remission of the inflammation with no evident loss of destruction resulting from it. Gingivitis may be physiological mechanisms that prevent – more than cause – the development of destructive periodontal diseases. The patient may develop periodontitis *despite* and not *because* of gingivitis. Thus it may not

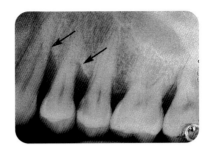

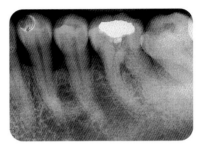

Fig 2 **Several forms of periodontal diseases** in the same mouth. Horizontal bone loss combined with areas where destruction is more rapid or has started earlier. (Arrows)

be feasible to treat mild gingivitis (unless periodontitis also is present). Moderate to severe cases of gingivitis, which causes discomfort to patients – or their surroundings – should of course be treated.

Periodontitis

Periodontitis is defined as a group of infectious diseases causing (irreversible?) destruction of the periodontal attachment, i.e. loss of alveolar bone and functional periodontal ligament. It is the loss of this attachment, observed clinically and roentgenologically, that reveals whether or not, and to what extent the patient has periodontitis. Bleeding on probing, edema and redness are other symptoms of periodontal inflammation (i.e. gingivitis).

Previously, gingivitis was regarded as an obligatory precursor for periodontitis. Modern periodontology regards gingivitis and periodontitis as two separate types of infections affecting the same area. The first is not destructive – the second is. However, it is difficult to find a periodontal lesion without the presence of gingivitis.

DIAGNOSIS OF PERIODONTITIS

All patients should be checked regularly for their periodontal condition, and the patient's record should be designed to accommodate the periodontal assessments and diagnosis.

A suggestion for a simple diagnostic system is presented at the end of this chapter. (page 29)

Plaque

The presence of plaque should be assessed in each approximal area, and on all lingual and buccal surfaces. This information is important for validation of the diagnosis and for preparing the motivation and oral hygiene instruction of the patient during the pre-treatment phase. In the future we will increasingly refer to plaque as the biofilm in order to describe this pathogenic biomass as a more vital object, than the use of the word plaque does.

Bleeding and suppuration

Gingival bleeding reflects inadequate plaque control and lack of collaboration. The presence or absence of gingival bleeding is, therefore, a highly relevant and important assessment.

Bleeding on probing (BOP) after careful probing to the *bottom* of the pocket with a blunt instrument, and/or pus from periodontal pockets, are frequently used to detect inflamed periodontal pockets. However, these measurements only suggest that there is inflammation present in the pocket and do not show that loss of attachment is ongoing. Thus BOP is not *a priori* an indication that destructive periodontitis is present. On the other hand, these symptoms suggest that there are objects of irritation in the pocket, and that they should be removed. The absence of bleeding on probing is on the other hand, in most cases, a clear indication of periodontal health.

The risk for periodontal destruction increases if the number of bleeding periodontal sites is high, (>30%) and if BOP continues over time.

Pocket measurement (Fig. 3)

Pocket measurement is the clinical parameter most often used in the diagnosis of periodontal diseases, and should be performed on mesial, buccal, distal and lingual aspects of all teeth. Pocket depth measurement is a quick way to get an overview of the patient's periodontal status. The measurement defined as the distance from the gingival margin to the bottom of the pocket, and reflects loss of attachment as well as increased height of the gingiva due to edema, hypertrophy or hyperplasia. To what extent this measurement represents actual loss of attachment, is not known, and may vary from patient to patient and between types of lesions. Pocket depth is thus a reasonable measurement for a point-in-time assessment in patients with little or no loss of attachment, but is less useful than clinical attachment level (CAL) (see below) in the monitoring of a patient before, during, and after treatment.

An important point when measuring pocket depth or loss of attachment (see below) with manual probes is not to apply more

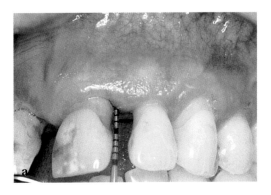
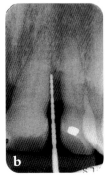

Fig 3 a,b
a. Pocket dept (PPD) and clinical attachment level(CAL) clinically measured with a blunt, graded periodontal probe
b. Roentgenogram of the same periodontal probe in the same position as in a.

that 20–25g pressure on the probe against the bottom of the pocket. By using too much pressure, one can force the probe through the pocket or junctional epithelium and into the underlying periodontal ligament, causing damage, pain and obviously incorrect measurement.

There are probes, both manual and computerized, that prevent the operator from using excessive force above 20g.

The periodontal attachment level
(Fig. 3)

The periodontal attachment level is defined as the distance from a fixed point, f. ex. the cemento-enamel junction, to the bottom of the pocket. **Loss of attachment** is a relative measurement that requires at least 2 measurements over time. This parameter of periodontal destruction has been more commonly used in research, but should be applied more in regular periodontal diagnostics than simple pocket depth measurements. Thus the attachment loss (2 measures of CAL over a period of time) reflects the speed with which the destruction has occurred, which is one of the objectives in diagnosis. Loss of attachment is the more suitable measurement for assessing treatment success and failure. When using loss of at-

tachment assessments, one should remember that due to restorative therapy, the cemento enamel junction (CEJ) may have been removed and with it, the reference point used in measuring loss of attachment. These measurements are also performed using periodontal probes with a pressure of 20 - 25g to the bottom of the pocket

Furcation involvement

Furcation involvement occurs in multirooted teeth where destruction of the alveolar bone has advanced to the point where there is opening into the area between roots. A furcation area has been suggested a risk site for further destruction, but may also quite frequently be a sign of pulpal involvement with communicating accessory channels between a necrotic – or partially necrotic – pulpal chamber and the interradical area. In this respect it is important to acknowledge that 20–25% of all multi-rooted teeth show accessory channels between the pulpa cavum and the interradical area. Assessment of furcation involvement is most easily done by probing with a curette. Furcation Grade I indicates that one can feel the entrance of the furcation; Grade II that one can probe partially through the furcation. In Grade III there is a trough-and-through passage between the roots.

Periodontal probes

There is a variety of periodontal probes on the market. Some are appropriately thin, with a blunt end to prevent the accidental penetration of the pocket epithelium. Others have a larger diameter all over. Some are color-coded, some are not.

The most recent manual periodontal probes have a disposable measuring part and an autoclavable handle (TPS Probe from VivaCare). This probe also has an additional design that prevents the use of excessive force beyond 20g.

It is of importance to use the same type of periodontal probe for the same patient before and after treatment, in order to evaluate treatment outcome. Also several automated periodontal probes have been marketed. The Florida probe and the Perioprobe contain computerized programs that recognize and digitalize the measurements made by the electronic probe, and prints them into a journal. The advantages of these probes are that they are more accurate, more reliable and save time and auxiliary personnel. Our experience is that the Florida probe is a research instrument, whereas the Perioprobe is more designed for everyday use in the clinic.

Voice-activated systems are also available, but are still very expensive. There are also automatized probes with a built-in ability to measure the temperature in the pocket. Increase in pocket temperature may, according to the manufacturer, precede a periodontal breakdown. The technique has, so far, attained scant attention in periodontal diagnostics.

The measurement errors of pocket and attachment loss measurements depend on the skills and experience of the operator as well as on the anatomical detail. The operator may, as stated above, use too much or too little force during measuring, and thereby over- or underestimate attachment loss or pocket depth. The tip of the probe may be prevented from reaching the bottom of the pocket by subgingival calculus or an irregularity of the root surface, resulting in incorrect measurement.

The American Academy of Periodontology (AAP) published a position paper (October 1996, Journal of Periodontology) on periodontal pocket/attachment loss measurements, in which it was stated, that: "the standard deviation of repeated manual pocket measurements is 0.8mm for a trained operator." **This means that the operator has to measure at least a 2mm change (2 standard deviations) in order to be sure that a true change in pocket depth/attachment level has occurred.**

In summary, we want to emphasize that although pocket depth and loss of attachment measurements depend on 'fingerspitzgefuhl' and dexterity, these are not by themselves sufficient for the complete diagnosis and monitoring of the periodontal condition or its treatment.

Roentgen diagnosis

Roentgen diagnosis is important as a supplement to clinical measurements. Vertical BiteWings are excellent for examination of the bone destruction in the posterior segments (Fig. 4). Using parallel technique, the operator may easily compare and evaluate bone destruction and treatment outcome over time. Orthopantomograms are so far not suitable for diagnosis or monitoring of periodontal conditions. This also goes for the digital OPGs claiming to have a "periodontal" modus. It still is too course to use as a diagnostic tool in periodontics.

Roentgenograms first and foremost show changes in the hard tissues. Neither X-rays nor clinical examination can show if a treatment has been successful in restoring periodontal ligament. Most commonly, periodontal treatment may result in bone growth

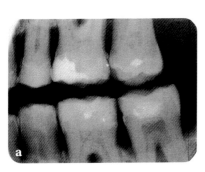
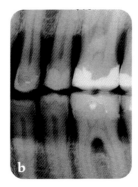
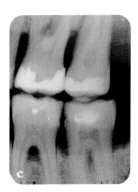

Fig 4 a – c Whereas horizontal bitewing roentgenograms (a) most frequently do not show the marginal bone , "standing" bitewing roentgenograms (b,c) are useful in diagnosing caries as well as qualitative diagnostics of the marginal bone.

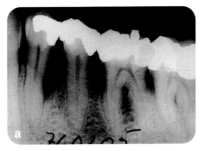
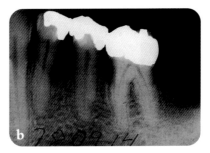

Fig 5 a,b Roentgenogram showing an infrabony pocket 34d, before – and 2 years after treatment.

against the previously affected root surface (Bone fill) (Fig. 5), and a long junctional epithelium between the root and the newly formed alveolar bone. X-rays will in such cases show increased roentgenographic bone mass and the clinical probing will indicate gain of attachment. All this despite the potential pocket between root and bone.

Tooth mobility

Tooth mobility may be a sign that the periodontal attachment is reduced, but also may indicate traumatic occlusion and an increased width of the periodontal ligament. Traumatic occlusion may be a modulating,

but not etiological factor, which makes the local situation seem more severe. Mobile teeth in an otherwise healthy, or slightly reduced periodontium, should make the operator look for malocclusion or interference (premature contacts).

Active or ongoing destruction

Active or ongoing destruction can only be detected by observing the patient over time. In a busy clinical practice the dentist must give priority to treatment of active periodontal disease, especially in young patients. It is not wrong to continue to monitor 'Mrs Smith' who first came to your practice in

1975 with some or several pockets of 4–5mm. The important thing is that the condition has been recorded based on ample diagnostic efforts. The continued monitoring of 'Mrs Smith' is quite acceptable because: a treated patient on a strict oral hygiene regimen faces reduced chances for further destruction.

Mechanical treatment as a diagnostic tool

A simple mild to moderate periodontal disease should be treated with scaling and root planing. It is of great importance that the instruments used are sharp, and share a design that favors the use in the different anatomical varied dentitions. *An adequate mechanical therapy most commonly results in the remission of the disease. Good oral hygiene prevents the return of the disease.* On the other hand, it is not uncommon to find continued destruction in patients with an adequate oral hygiene and who have had scaling and root planing. The recurrence of disease may be generalized, or only confined to a few teeth. Frequently, destruction in these patients commences so fast that one may regard the disease as a rapidly destructive periodontitis.

We have already acknowledged that several types of periodontitis may exist in the same mouth, and that the slowly destructive periodontitis may mask the rapidly destructive type, because the first is much more common then the latter. In addition, both types of infections display the same combination of symptoms. *In such cases we should use the mechanical treatment as a diagnostic tool to identify the more serious rapidly destructive periodontal disease.*

By using conventional mechanical treatment it is possible to eliminate the non-specific, slowly progressing periodontitis, by eliminating the cause of the infection, i.e. the subgingival dental biofilm (plaque) and calculus. Subsequently one is left with pockets with 'specific infections' that do not respond to this 'non-specific therapy'.

In the past there was a tendency to call these periodontal diseases refractory or treatment resistant periodontal diseases. However what may be a refractory periodontal disease to one clinician, may perhaps be treated successfully by another. Is it then refractory? Our view is that *refractory periodontitis is a periodontitis that has not received adequate treatment, or received the wrong diagnosis!*

MICROBIOLOGICAL DIAGNOSIS

Having diagnosed destructive periodontal disease, instructed the patient in meticulous oral hygiene, and even treated the disease 'by the book' with conventional mechanical therapy, we occasionally are confronted with patients or single sites that continue to break down, and where conventional mechanical treatment has failed. The most common reason for this 'refractory disease' is a patient's lack of meticulous oral hygiene, or insufficient scaling and root planing. Another possibility is that one is dealing with an infection, which cannot be cured mechanically. This is what may be regarded as a 'specific infection'. If one is absolutely certain that both the oral hygiene and the mechanical treatment have been adequate, one should introduce specific diagnostic approaches in order to ascertain the nature of the infection, so that the treatment plan can be revised. Over the last decade there has been a growing interest in microbial testing as part of the diagnosis and treatment planning of periodontal disease. Increased focus on the role of specific infection in the etiology of some destructive periodontal diseases and in cases of transmission of periodontal diseases has revealed a hidden demand for expanded diagnostics.

Today, laboratories all over the world pro-

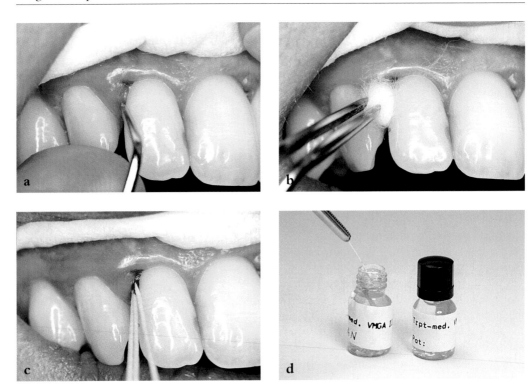

Fig 6 a – d Microbiological diagnosis. a) Supragingival debris is being removed by curettes. b) The tooth surface is cleaned with a sterile cotton pellet, c) 1–3 sterile paper points (Medium size) are placed at the bottom of the pocket(s) d) After 10 sec., the paper points are removed and subsequently placed in the transport medium. The sample is sent to the laboratory with a specific form detailing name and vital data of the patient and the sampling. (Photos: Dr Lars Sjöström)

vide microbiological diagnostic services for dentists. Our experience is that one should not use general medical laboratories, but rather collaborate with laboratories run by microbiologists knowledgeable in oral microbiology. Many university laboratories, those associated with dental schools, provide such services.

If you want to start using laboratory tests (Fig. 6) in your practice, you should ask the designated laboratory for test tubes containing transport medium, padded envelopes and the forms necessary to go with the bacterial sample. The indication for microbial testing is that your patient has a rapidly destructive periodontal disease that is not ar-

rested by adequate mechanical treatment and a well-performed oral hygiene. The clinician should select the pockets that he wants to sample, remove the supragingival plaque or debris, air-dry the area, and insert one ore more sterile paper points to the bottom of the pocket. After 10 seconds, the points are removed and immediately inserted into the transport medium. The tube is carefully closed, the form is completed with relevant patient data and disease information, and the sample(s) forwarded to the laboratory.

In the laboratory, the samples are seeded on different media for culturing, or processed for gene probing or other, if such methods are available. After 7–14 days the laboratory will return the results of the tests, e.g., the amount of the different bacteria present and a resistance profile of the suspected pathogen(s). With this information, together with all the other data obtained of the disease and the patient, the clinician may now develop a treatment plan for the individual patient. This approach has proved very useful in cases of rapidly progressing periodontal disease as well as for evaluating potential or real risks for transmission between family members or other.

A microbial test does not provide the full diagnosis of the disease, but allows for additional information that may or may not be useful in selecting treatment strategies in different cases. Selection of strategies in periodontal disease control will be discussed in depth later in this book.

However, before considering microbiological testing or establishing treatment strategies, it is imperative that all other possible reasons for the observed conditions are ruled out.

DIFFERENTIAL DIAGNOSIS

There are periodontal conditions that display symptoms almost identical to those of periodontal disease, without actually being periodontitis. In such cases a treatment strategy aimed at treating periodontal disease will not be useful. Consequently a thorough differential diagnosis must be made.

Periapical ostitis (Fig. 7)

Periapical ostitis may have established a fistula-like channel within the periodontal membrane proper and empties its content at the gingival margin, thereby creating an illusion of a periodontal pocket. Normally, a fistula heals after removal of its cause. How-

ever, mechanical treatment of this condition, as if it were periodontal disease, will evidently reduce the possibilities of healing the fistula. Only endodontic treatment will make the condition heal, depending on how long the condition has existed, and to what degree a superimposed periodontal disease component has added to the clinical situation. Therefore, it is important to have this possibility in mind and to rule out such conditions by high quality X-rays. One should be especially alert when suddenly discovering a very deep periodontal pocket in an otherwise periodontally healthy dentition.

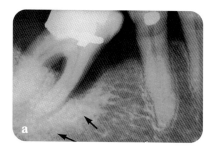

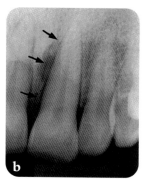

Fig 7 a,b Examples of periodontal destruction caused primarily by endodontic problems. a) a necrotic pulpal channel in the mesial root of a tilted 47 may be faultily diagnosed as a periodontal pocket. Proper endodontic treatment will cause new attachment, whereas a primary periodontal scaling and root planing will inevitably result in the loss of attachment as far down as the lower 1/3 of the root. b) A mesial bony defect on 21, caused by a necrotic pulp and an accessory root canal in the lower 1/3 of the root.

Deep periodontal pockets do not develop overnight!

Fistulas are narrow on probing, whereas periodontal, infrabony pockets are clinically wider.

Root fractures (Figs. 8 and 9)

Root fractures are solitary conditions that may look like refractory periodontal diseases on single teeth. One should be especially observant in endodontically treated teeth, with or without restorations. High-quality X-rays, obtained from different angles, may provide the answers but sometimes only explorative surgery will reveal the fractures – often, hidden on X-rays by pulpal pins, screws, or endodontic material.

Enamel projections

Enamel projections at the lingual aspect of incisors or laterals in the upper jaw, as well as in the buccal entrance to bifurcations of molars of the lower jaw are not uncommon. Occurrence of solitary pockets in these same locations may present different diagnostic problems. One cannot evaluate a lesion like that before the enamel projection is removed through grinding and a 3–6 months period has elapsed in order to give time for new attachment, or further deepening of the pocket. However, these are not diseases, only physiological pockets with gingivitis, and thus normally only subject to assessment of destruction during routine controls.

Drug-related gingival hyperplasia (Fig. 10)

Drug-related gingival hyperplacia is most commonly caused by the use of Fenytoin, Cyclosporins and Calcium antagonists. It is

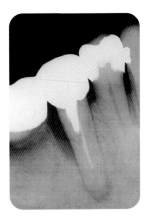

Fig 8 Horizontal root fracture with vertical periodontal destruction. (Photos; Drs. E.Haugen and J.R.Johansen)

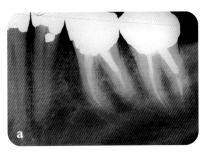

Fig 9 a Roentgenogram of a wide and deep infrabony pocket mesial to 36.

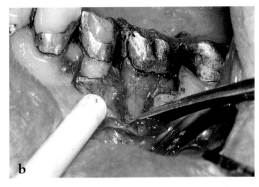

Fig 9 b Following flap surgery a vertical root fracture appears explaining the local bone destruction.

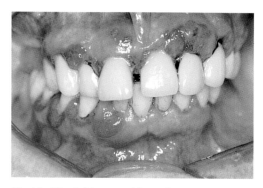

Fig 10 Gingivitis caused by a Ca-antagonist.

important to obtain an accurate history from the patient in order to make a diagnosis of this disease. Meticulous oral hygiene in such cases is essential.

Pregnancy gingivitis

Pregnancy gingivitis often looks like chronic periodontitis due to the edematous increase in the width of the periodontal membrane. Misdiagnosis often results during the first trimester, when the pregnancy is not evident to the therapist. The most commonly involved teeth are the molars, and clinically one observes increased mobility, measurable periodontal pockets, and bleeding on prob-

ing. True pregnancy gingivitis will heal *post partum*, but in the past resulted in a disturbing number of extractions

Estrogen gingivitis

Estrogen gingivitis is a possible diagnosis observed occasionally in women who are administered Estrogen for their menopausal discomfort. The most common observation is a quite severe gingivitis and pseudopockets, which resemble chronic periodontitis. A normal, good oral hygiene does not seem to help, and the patients are quite often anxious because of the bleeding. Most patients experience relief from the condition by improving their standard of oral hygiene, but may also discuss the problem with their physician who might reduce the dosage or change to another drug brand. We have also occasionally seen possible reaction to hormonal contraceptives of other kinds.

Root remnants from the deciduous dentition (Fig. 11)

Root remnants from the deciduous dentition are rare phenomena, but may resemble

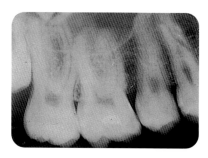
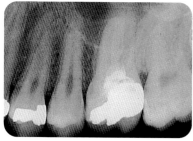

Fig 11 Remains of deciduous root 16m and an infected pulpal inlay in 26 caused respectively a 6mm pocket 16m and a 7mm pocket 26d. This clinical find in a 17 year old boy led to the faulty diagnosis of Localized Juvenile Periodontitis, which after closer examination turned out to be a double differential diagnosis. Both defects healed spontaneously after removal of the deciduous root juxtapositioned to 16 and revision of endodontic filling 26.

calculus on root surfaces when projected over the roots on roentgenograms.

RISK FACTORS

Diseases and conditions predisposing for periodontal disease

Risk factors are systemic diseases, hormonal changes, personal behavior or lifestyle, environmental factors or inherited characteristics, which in epidemiological studies are observed previous to, and have a causal relationship with, the development of periodontal disease.

Periodontal disease is an infection caused by bacteria, which leads to the tooth gradually losing its supporting tissue. The loss of attachment is mostly irreversible. There are many known and unknown risk factors, which can interact in the development and progression of this destructive infection. Knowledge about these risk factors enables clinicians to categorize and individualize the specific periodontal infection, and thus more easily select an effective treatment strategy.

It is therefore important to realize that there are several periodontal diseases, and that by categorizing disease and symptoms together with risk factor and cause-analysis, it is possible to individualize the view of the diseases and to choose an individualized diagnosis and treatment. The 'scaling for all' approach is no longer an acceptable concept.

Familial aggregation of periodontal disease – transmission

One reason for familial aggregation of periodontal disease is that the oral bacterial flora is transmitted from parents to children. The primary role of specific bacteria in the development of periodontal disease is now widely accepted. Bacteria like *A. actinomycetemcomitans, P. gingivalis,* spirochetes and other are involved in the pathogenesis; they are present in high numbers in periodontal diseases, but are absent or found in low numbers in periodontal health. These bacteria produce potent virulence factors, and may also provoke specific immune reactions. Even though there is an association between these bacteria and disease, this is no simple cause-relationship. Also, even though there are several bacterial species present in the periodontal pocket, only *A. actinomycetemcomitans* and *P. gingivalis* have been studied in greater detail.

From Dr. Preus and coworkers' own studies, it seems as if *A. actinomycetemcomitans* in families where one of the parents suffers from periodontal disease, transmits from adults to children. Dr. Preus found that transmission between spouses or cohabitants was rare or absent. The reason for this is, perhaps, that *A. actinomycetemcomitans* does not easily invade and colonize an already established oral flora, because it is rejected by oral streptococci in general and *S. sanguis* in particular. *A. actinomycetemcomitans* seems to establish itself in the oral flora in periods of general microbiological change. The shedding of deciduous teeth and establishing of the permanent dentition cause a change in the oral flora where any microorganism may colonize a niche. At the same time, and as a consequence of the changes in the dentition, there is serum available. *A. actinomycetemcomitans* needs serum in order to colonize and grow.

It is also possible that hormonal factors, which appear in the mouth during puberty, may assist in facilitating the colonization process for this organism. With reference to these observations we assume that *A. actinomycetemcomitans* establishes itself in the period of early puberty. Later establishment is also possible, but is probably uncommon. If it happens, it will be in periods of changes in the oral flora. F.ex. during general malaise, following antibiotic therapy or during other infections when the oral flora is in 'turmoil'. In families where one or more family members suffers from Localized advanced Periodontitis in young adults, see appendix (LAY – Also called Localized Juvenile Periodontitis [LJP]), Dr. Preus' studies showed that the A. actinomycetemcomitans clone(s) isolated from active sites in LAY/LJP patients were also most frequently found in one of the parents. These studies also indicated that, depending on living conditions, the bacterial transmission originated outside the family, and that in some cases this infection was truly an exogenous infection.

An entirely new idea is also that LAY/LJP may not be a true periodontal disease, but rather an ostitis, juxtapositioned to the periodontal membrane. This idea is based on the observation that LAY/LJP patients regained their lost periodontium solely through the use of antibiotic therapy. Also we observed on X-rays that LAY lesions were often droplet-shaped, with a rounded base below the most apical point in the periodontal membrane, but a short distance therefrom indicating that the destruction center is within the interproximal bone and "affecting or reaching" the periodontal membrane secondarily like "ripples in a pond". These observations indicate another primary treatment for this disease entity than other periodontitis diagnosis, which we will discuss in detail later.

The relationship of P. gingivalis to the periodontal syndrome is somewhat less complicated. Studies show that the transmission of this bacterium occurs between all family members regardless of age. This might not be surprising since P. gingivalis seems to thrive in subgingival dental plaque, and does not experience the same resistance against its establishment as do A. actinomycetemcomitans. On the other hand, it is said that P. gingivalis is found only in patients with established periodontal disease, and that only patients with disease may act as donors for the spread of this organism. It is not known how frequently such transmission occurs, but it has been suggested that as soon as a clone of P. gingivalis has colonized a person's mouth, it will immediately spread to the rest of the family.

Some researchers have characterized periodontal disease as a 'kissing disease', inferring that periodontal microorganisms might be transmitted through kissing. Such statements put periodontal disease in a class with other transmittable diseases. Such statements cause fear and anxiety among people, are unnecessary, and plainly wrong. There is no evidence whatsoever that acquiring a clone of A. actinomycetemcomitans or P. gingivalis will eventually lead to disease. Nor are the patterns of transmission and incubation time anywhere close to those of the common transmissible diseases. On the other hand, colonization by these bacteria is quite commonly associated with the experience of periodontal disease. Therefore, the causal relationship is not as clear as some researchers want to believe, although the presence of these organisms in the subgingival biofilm is a risk factor. Our view is that these oral bacteria are acquired through the normal buildup of the individual's microbial flora. It is based on sheer unluck that one acquire a pathogenic periodontal microorganism because one of the parents (or other frequent donors) carries such bacteria, and thus acquires a higher risk for developing periodontal disease.

Systemic conditions/diseases – risk factors.

Systemic conditions are defined as naturally occurring or induced conditions, which will affect the whole host organism. They may be hormonal, nutritional, genetic, age-related, or drugs such as the use of tobacco, the environment, or stress.

Age

Most populations show increased periodontal disease with increased age, but there is no clear indication as to how age *per se* may influence the progression of periodontal disease. On the contrary, studies have shown that, corrected for the level of oral hygiene, age is a weak 'risk factor' in the development of periodontal disease.

The increased frequency of periodontitis in the elderly may have more to do with the fact that oral hygiene procedures grow increasingly difficult with growing age, due to physical, and mental limitations. *P. gingivalis* may be more common in the elderly. *P. gingivalis* and *A. actinomycetemcomitans* are pathogens often associated with periodontal destruction. On the other hand, the elderly are mostly as efficient as younger people in producing antibodies against infectious challenges, and there are no indications that aging per se weakens the organism thereby allowing periodontal disease to develop. **Actually, it seems that disease in the elderly is a consequence of an accumulation of destruction, or symptoms, due to periodontitis experiences over a lifetime**.

Race

Race has commonly been associated with the frequency of periodontal disease in a population. Previous studies indicated that African Americans had more periodontal disease than Caucasians. More recent studies show that when African Americans are selected from the same socio-economic group as Caucasians, there is no difference in the frequency of periodontal diseases. This indicates that socio-economic status and related factors, such as education and the use of dental services are more related to the presence of periodontal diseases than race *per se*. This has been confirmed in studies showing that 46% of all African Americans and 16% of all whites in the same age group had periodontal disease, but that socio-economic factors were pivotal in the development and severity of the disease. Also, the studies showed that there were differences in periodontal microbiology between African American and whites, in the sense that the former group had more *A. actinomycetemcomitans* and *P. gingivalis* in their oral flora. Thus, it is concluded that race is not a risk factor for periodontal diseases, but rather that the race is associated with microbiological as well as other – less defined – differences.

Socio-economic and nutritional status

Several Scandinavian researchers have studied socio-economic and nutritional status. Pindborg found that men with higher socio-economic status had healthier periodontium than those with lower. Arno et al. showed similar results when they compared the periodontal situation in supervisors and workers in the same factories; and Løvdal showed that it was neither income nor economical status but educational level that was the deciding factor. It is also clear that there are large differences in the presence of periodontal diseases in industrialized and developing countries, with more disease in the latter. The differences have been attributed to nutritional status, but it has been shown that neither vitamin deficiency nor shortage of essentials like keratinin, thiamin, riboflavin, or methylnicotinamid have any impact on the development of periodontal diseases.

Diabetes mellitus

In a study of the Pima Indians in the USA 20 years ago, Genco et al. observed large differences in the prevalence of periodontal disease between those who suffered from diabetes mellitus and those that did not. When corrections where made for hygiene, age, gender, smoking, etc., there was still an association between diabetes mellitus and periodontal disease. Also, the incidence of periodontal disease was accelerated (2.5x) in diabetes patients than in those of the healthy controls. These observations strengthen the suggested association between the two diseases. Studies have thus suggested that changes in the capillary wall, defective neutrophils and/or specific microbiology in diabetes patients may alone, or in combination, be responsible for the association. Recent research indicate that there are certain common immunological mediators in both diseases, which increase the severity of each other in addition to the increased severity of the disease proper.

Poorly controlled diabetes is strongly associated with the development of periodontitis, whereas a well-maintained and controlled diabetes patient is as easy (or difficult) to treat as a non-diabetic. On the other hand, a severe case of periodontitis, as any other severe infection, makes it difficult to select and maintain the insulin dosage necessary to control the diabetes. Thus, there is a two-way association between diabetes and periodontal disease, both in this respect, and as mentioned above. This makes it even more important to diagnose and effectively treat periodontal disease in these patients.

Pregnancy and sex hormones

These have been described under Differential Diagnoses, and we do not regard these as risk factors for destructive periodontal diseases, only for gingivitis.

Down's syndrome

An association between the presence of trisomy 21 and periodontitis has been described in the literature. This association cannot be explained by insufficient oral hygiene. Studies are in progress to investigate if specific bacteriology or changed leukocytes may account for this association.

Other, rare diseases

HIV/AIDS has often been associated with changes in gingival tissues (Fig. 12). HIV gingivitis, necrotic periodontitis and Kaposi's sarcoma are conditions that must be recognized by the clinician even if the occurrence is rather rare. Acute Necrotizing Ulcerative Gingivitis/Periodontitis (ANUG/P) should today be regarded as a condition that may be associated to HIV/AIDS. The diagnosis of ANUG should therefore always arouse suspicion of HIV/AIDS. This should be followed up by appropriate investigation.

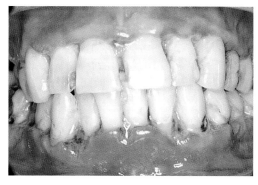

Fig 12 Acute Necrotizing Ulcerating Gingivitis (ANUG) in a HIV positive patient.

Patients with abnormally functioning granulocytes, like in neutropenia, in reduced adherence and chemotaxis, or oncogenic changes (e.g. as in leukemia) often show changes that bring to mind ulcerations rather more than periodontal diseases.

Stress and periodontal diseases

Studies have shown associations between stress and periodontal diseases. Recent studies by Dr Breivik et al. indicate that the association with periodontal diseases is caused by changes in the host response to infectious challenges and not only to stress related habits. Sudden onset of gingivitis and/or periodontitis should launch a thorough investigation into the patient's psychosocial relations (divorce, death, disease in nearest family, etc.). It is a known fact that the immunological system reacts inadequately as a result of prolonged episodes of sleeplessness, hunger and in periods of depression. Today, the implications of stress in the pathogenesis of periodontal diseases are interesting fields of research.

Tobacco related implications

Recent studies indicate that the use of tobacco is a clear risk factor in the pathogenesis of periodontitis. The risk for developing periodontitis is 3–5 times higher in smokers than in non-smokers. Whereas chewing tobacco may cause ulcerations and cancer, smoking tobacco is normally associated with periodontal disease. It seems that smokers have a more complex, and severe periodontitis than non-smokers, and the discovery of periodontal pockets on the palatal sites of the upper jaw is commonly seen for smokers' periodontitis. Studies have shown that 90% of all recurring cases of periodontal disease were attributable to smokers. However, the causal relation is not yet clear. However, it has been suggested that smokers are:

1. Less careful when performing their daily oral hygiene, and thus exhibit higher plaque scores than non-smokers
2. More exposed to oral anaerobic bacteria than non-smokers due to less oxygen tension in their mouths, and
3. More exposed to nicotine-related constriction of the gingival blood vessels, causing an imbalance between reparative and destructive forces in the periodontal pathogenesis.

Both 1 and 2 above has been refuted in controlled studies, leaving us with the last explanation, which also appears to be the most logical one. Cause-effect relations have not been found in this context, though.

Genetic aspects

Is there a predisposition for the development of periodontal disease? And if so, is it inheritable? In Localized Aggressive Periodontitis = localized advanced young (LAY) (see p 29) the disease has an autosomal recessive inheritance, leaving the patients with a reduced capacity for neutrophil chemotaxis. There is no definite research linking LAY to HLA antigens. However, recent research has suggested a genetic predisposition in the development of periodontal disease, and a test that claims to single out those patients at risk to develop periodontal disease is in the offing.

The release of prostaglandin is essential in the pathogenesis of periodontal disease. This is triggered by certain cytokines, i.e. IL1β, and is suggested to be genetically regulated. A diagnostic kit for identification of this specific polymorphism of IL1β has been developed, and is being tested clinically. Tobacco smoking tends to mask the effect of this IL1β.

Association between periodontitis and other diseases or conditions

Lately Periodontitis has been associated with Coronary Heart Disease, stroke and pre-term birth. Epidemiological studies have shown a high degree of common factors that could explain the association, but no causal relationship has been established. Therefore, several hypotheses have been put forward to explain such possible causal relationship, of which those claiming common immuno-logical mediators for the different traits have been the most popular. However, given time, several thorough Random Controlled Clinical Trials (RCTs) have been reported recently, and these suggest no such associa-tion. Therefore, these intriguing associa-tions seems unclear, and we must wait for further research before we involve ourselves in changing clinical behavior and approach-es due to this.

In summary it may be concluded that the greatest risk factors for the development of periodontal disease are:

1. Insufficient oral hygiene
2. Presence of specific periodontal path-ogens
3. Diabetes mellitus, type I
4. Smoking of more than 10 cigarettes per day, and
5. Stress.

Diagnosis of Periodontits

Lately a series of different ways to diagnose and classify periodontal diseases have been presented in he literature. We feel that the nominative description of the disease at hand gives the most information to the clinician, and suggest to use the below described sys-tem for diagnosing periodontal diseases in the clinic.

The system is based on 3 different charac-teristics of the disease
1. The number of teeth involved (spread of infection)
2. How serious these defects are (Clinical loss of attachment CAL)
3. The age of the patient

In addition we add a description of special features about the disease or the patient (Acute, Chronic, Rapidly progressive, Bac-terial diagnosis, etc), or moderating circum-stances like general diseases (diabetes) that may affect the expression of the periodontal disease.

1. Classification based on the number of teeth involved:
Localized disease (1-7 teeth)
Generalised (>7 teeth)

2. Classification based on seriousness:
No – or slight disease: Does not apply to moderate (2) or serious (3)
Moderate: At least 2 teeth with LA>1/3, but <1/2 of the length of the root (x-ray), or CAL >3 mm, but <5mm.
Advanced (serious): At least 2 teeth with LA >1/2 of the length of the root (x-ray), or CAL >5mm.

3. Classification based on age (at last birthday):
Young: ≤ 30 years-of-age.
Adult: >30 years-of-age

This will together give 3 criteria with which to label the disease at hand.

Example:
GMA = Generalized, Moderate, Adult (diabetic).
LAY = Localized, Advanced, Young,
LAY = Localized, Advanced, Young (15 Years, A. actinomycetemcomitans)

CHAPTER 2

Initial Therapy – Patient Management

Comprehensive treatment strategy

The keys to successful treatment of periodontal disease are:

Knowledge
about the epidemiology, etiology and pathogenesis of periodontal diseases, their treatment and prevention

Structure
in the management and treatment strategy of patients with periodontal disease in accordance with individual patient's needs

High quality
in patient care and treatment, and

Dedication
to success.

Steps in the comprehensive strategy in the management of periodontal patients are:

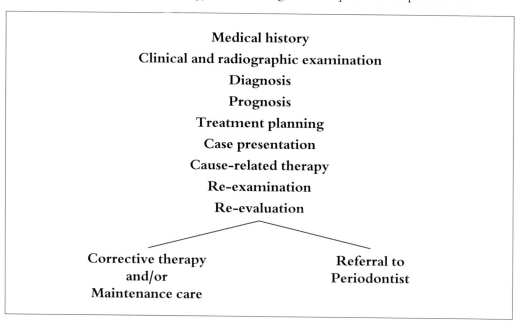

Medical history
Clinical and radiographic examination
Diagnosis
Prognosis
Treatment planning
Case presentation
Cause-related therapy
Re-examination
Re-evaluation

Corrective therapy and/or Maintenance care

Referral to Periodontist

It is the dental practitioner who is responsible for the care of the patient. Some of the elements in this structure such as the clinical examination and cause-related therapy can be performed by a dental hygienist, but the dentist is at the end of the day responsible for the diagnosis, the prognosis and the treatment planning. The dental practitioner should also make the re-evaluation, and determine the further treatment strategy.

Prognosis

Following clinical and radiographic examination and diagnosis a prognosis should be made for:

Every single tooth
The entire dentition
Treatment outcome on a short-term and long-term basis.

If advanced periodontal disease is diagnosed, one or several teeth may have to be extracted because they cannot be successfully treated – their prognosis is poor or bad. Other teeth may have a questionable prognosis. These are important factors to consider at an early stage, and should be included in the case presentation prior to active treatment. Teeth that are untreatable should be extracted as soon as possible since they constitute a risk/source for re-infection of treated areas. When required, extracted teeth should be replaced with temporary fixed or removable prosthetic appliances. Final prosthetic appliances should not be contemplated until the patient is successfully treated and considered periodontally healthy, which includes an observational period of several months or further

Treatment planning

Following detailed examination and diagnosis an appropriate treatment plan is made and presented to the patient. It is important that this includes short-term and final treatment goals. These must be understood and accepted by the patient, so that the patient can assume a partner's responsibility in the treatment of the disease. Thus, he is now able to follow the development towards a healthy outcome.

Treatment

Cause-related periodontal therapy includes:
– Information to the patient about the disease and motivation
– Instruction in adequate, disease-related oral hygiene, and
– Elimination of the supra- and sub-gingival infection.

The initial, cause-related therapies are basically non-surgical, but may also include surgical elements, if considered necessary to accomplish the elimination of sub-gingival infection. The therapist's knowledge, clinical skill and experience are crucial factors in the treatment outcome.

Re-evaluation

The outcome of therapy should be evaluated by clinical (and radiographic when appropriate) examination following each step in the treatment plan to ascertain that the defined treatment goals are achieved (See Chapter 6). The results of the re-evaluation should be used to design further corrective and/or supportive treatment, or as a basis for referring the patient to a periodontist for specialist care.

Periodontal disease categories

In order to design the proper treatment strategy, it may be beneficial/practical to divide periodontal diseases into two major categories: the moderate (chronic, slowly progressive), and the severe (rapidly progressive) (see page 29). Chronic periodontitis is caused by non-specific infections and can easily be prevented and treated in its early stages through non-surgical means. Severe (rapidly progressive) periodontitis, on the other hand, usually has a complex etiology and pathogenesis, and requires special attention and knowledge to be successfully treated. Consequently patients with aggressive periodontitis ought to be referred to a periodontist.

Placing each case in the right category helps us to arrive at the correct diagnosis and a reasoned prognosis, as well as providing the effective treatment of these diseases, which Dr Roy Page once called "a family of related diseases that differ in etiology, natural history disease progression and response to therapy, but have a common chain of events."

One prerequisite for a successful treatment of a patient with periodontitis is that the treatment and the following supportive care should be adjusted according to the patient's intellectual resources.

Oral hygiene

The specific and the non-specific infection hypotheses as explained in Chapter 1, can be used to explain the clinical picture that we see in our patients. It has become gradually obvious that the degree of destruction of the periodontal tissues in periodontitis is not related to the amount of supra-gingival bacterial plaque.

Nevertheless, good oral hygiene is of paramount importance both in the treatment and prevention of periodontal disease in the non-specific as well as in the specific infection model. In the non-specific model the sub-gingival microbial biofilm with its billions of different microorganisms represents a collective risk for developing periodontal diseases. The more bacteria there are in the biofilm the higher the risk for the presence of pathogenic microorganisms. The more plaque, the higher the risk for microorganisms to spread to other areas. Consequently, a high standard of oral hygiene is mandatory for a successful periodontal treatment, whether the disease is considered a non-specific or a specific infection.

In Chapter 1 we referred to epidemiological studies, which have demonstrated that periodontitis may be found in 50% or more of the adult population. Knowledgeable practitioners can prevent this from developing by:
- Making early diagnosis
- Instituting preventive measures, including improved oral hygiene
- Starting early high-quality treatment, or
- Referring the patient to a periodontist where necessary.

Despite efforts to maintain patients with a high level of oral health, new patients with severe periodontal disease will show up. This may initially cause some disturbance in the routine of the practice. However, in a longer perspective a practitioner with good knowledge in diagnosis, treatment and prevention of periodontal disease will have a large patient list with periodontally healthy patients, and only a small fraction of patients who need extra attention and care because of severe periodontal disease.

Cases of severe advanced periodontal disease create uncertainties in other areas of every day practice. Periodontal treatment is technically demanding as well as resource and time consuming, and the general practitioner may not have the necessary time to arrive at successful treatment outcomes. There is also an economic issue here, since it may be difficult to charge the patient for just 'discussion and instruction'. Patients may not feel that they are paying for 'services rendered'.

It is, therefore, important to develop the attitude that your knowledge and expertise is worth something, in much the same way as knowledge and expertise of a lawyer, a family therapist, a psychiatrist or a financial adviser are financially esteemed. You have to learn to charge your patients for your services like other professionals do. Your fee is a reasonable compensation for *the knowledge you are prepared to share* with the patient. This may, however, be difficult for the patient to accept, unless the patient is informed and made to understand that knowledge is the key to successful disease prevention and treatment, and that knowledge has a price!

At the same time, this is part of the motivational effort, and the less time that needs to be spent on motivating and instructing the patient, the less expensive the whole treatment becomes. Oral hygiene is part of the total personal hygiene, and good oral hygiene contributes to the entire health and well-being. Thus, the dentist actually plays an important role in general healthcare.

Patient motivation

Patient motivation aims at, making the patient realize that he or she has a periodontal condition and that it is his or her role and responsibility to comply with given instructions. Successful treatment of periodontal disease is also highly dependent on the therapist's (dentist or dental hygienist) ability to establish a good communication with the patient. It is of the utmost importance that following the case presentation; the patient understands his/her situation and that both partial and final goals of the treatment are clearly defined. This initial part of the relationship is crucial and must be allocated the time necessary. A good idea is to either set up sufficient time for these appointments or to schedule these patients at the end of the day, when there is less 'time pressure'. This will allow for a better dialog, and leave time for all the questions the patient wants to have answered.

To be able to motivate a patient, it is necessary to have a good knowledge about the disease, its prevention and treatment, and to be able to transfer this knowledge to the patient by individualizing the information. The therapists' self-confidence, belief in themselves and their knowledge and ability, as well as their dedication to the task are important ingredients for success.

Very often practitioners act as if the patient knows more about oral disease and dental care than is actually the case, and takes 'short cuts' in the information process. The fact is that the average patient **knows very little** about dental care. We usually grow up with tooth brushing without really giving it a thought. The toothbrush may be moved around in the mouth twice daily without really accomplishing much plaque removal. To break this behavior, and to make oral hygiene practices effective, the patient must be taught a proper disease-related oral hygiene. Knowledge is the only means to reach this goal, and we have to create a patient's need to seek this knowledge. This need may be created by e.g. asking the patient about his or her attitude to the disease, knowledge and prejudice. Such a dialog will undoubtedly create *confidence* in the practitioner, arouse *curiosity about the situation,* and *generate motivation* to find a solution to the problems.

If the patient cannot see or understand the problem, there is little hope of having a motivated patient, and a poor treatment outcome may be expected. On the other hand, a casual comment about areas needing better cleaning while you are probing the pockets is meaningless, and will have little impact. The patient is just waiting for the probing to hurt, is tense and worried, and will not absorb the information on offer.

The motivation process should consist of information about the disease, its cause and development in the short and in the long term, its treatment and prevention. The patient should understand what habits and factors may influence the disease progression, such as genetic, local and environmental factors (e.g. susceptibility, diabetes, smoking, etc.) but also the implication of therapy. The therapist has to discover the patient's true disposition and attitude. Does the patient really understand the problem? Does the patient really believe that something can be done? Or has he or she heard too many stories about failures to trust you?

Remember: *the outcome of the individual motivation process will to a large extent determine the overall treatment outcome.*

Communication technique

To obtain the best possible dialog, the patient should be given a comfortable chair that he or she can more or less control (Fig. 13). Also, this should preferably be in a relaxed atmosphere (which is ideally not a treatment room). A patient on his back in a supine position in a dental chair will feel unsafe, uncomfortable and defenseless. A patient in such a position is not receptive to information. This position is actually meant for treatment and submission, not for dialog, motivation and instruction. Face to face communication is facilitated in the upright position. In this position the patient will feel more on the same level as the therapist.

Once a good contact has been obtained, the dentist or dental hygienist can start explaining the disease; that it is an infectious disease caused by bacteria that destroy the tissues, thereby creating a periodontal pocket where bacteria can hide and develop a microbiological community that will cause continued tissue destruction, and eventually loss of the tooth. It is extremely important that the patient does not feel ashamed or guilty, as this may obstruct or even block further communication. Make the patient realize that *periodontitis is an infectious disease*. Pro-

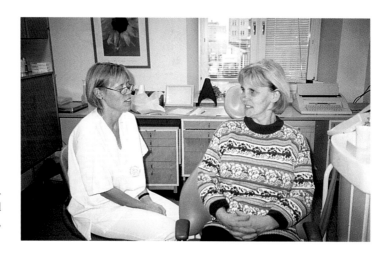

Fig 13 Correct communication between patient and therapist. Both sitting up, talking to each other

viding this part of the information may not take very long, but the information has to be given on the patient's own terms and in ways that the patient will understand. And even more important, if you can provide something that the patient did not know, or has not understood from previous information provided by another dentist, you will be able to establish and build growing trust and confidence. A small pamphlet that compliments the verbal instruction should be given to the patient. However, even if you are a good teacher, the patient may not remember everything you said. So reading the pamphlet may be their homework before the next appointment. A pamphlet may also be considered as material the patient 'purchased'. People are used to pay for reading material, and appreciate the work that has gone into its production. So, for different reasons, the written information pamphlet is an important 'extra' in the communication process.

Oral hygiene instructions

This part of the treatment should start with a comprehensive description of the tooth anatomy and how tooth cleaning is best performed. Based on the foregoing information the patient knows a good deal about periodontal disease, etiology treatment and prevention. In addition, as a therapist you know the patient's situation and treatment needs, as well as the patient's knowledge and attitude. So you can now design your instructions based on the patient's needs. Good instructions demand creativity, imagination and individualization. For example, you have to tell the patient that the tooth has four surfaces and how these are located. To do this you need a model of a tooth and a jaw. You can also use your fists or anything that can resemble a tooth. Preferably use two fists to illustrate their relationship and the interproximal spaces. This simplifies the whole

process. Then repeat the instructions in the patient's own mouth and show what interproximal spaces are. When the patient becomes aware of the fact that these areas are the main sites for periodontitis, it is also easy to understand that cleaning between teeth is important, and will require another 'tool' than the normal tooth brush. In fact the patient will realize that interproximal cleaning is the most important part in the prevention and treatment of periodontitis. Consequently a disease-related tooth cleaning procedure should start with the cleaning between teeth. Continue lingually and then finish with buccal brushing. Breaking old, insufficient habits will be beneficial for developing new and adequate habits. Excessive buccal gingival recession and attachment loss has occurred because of over-intensive buccal tooth-brushing. One properly performed tooth cleaning procedure per day is likely to be sufficient, and may be done at anytime of the day.

Conventional information and instructions that practitioners give their patients are not always taken in by patients, either because the instructions are too authoritarian, or do not allow for individualization and understanding. As we stressed above, it is important that you understand that patient knowledge is a prerequisite for optimal patient compliance. Knowledge is the only way to success, and information techniques are the vehicle by which to reach the goal. The direct instruction should always be a two-way communication, a dialog. Finally, do always follow up your information and instructions with regular plaque controls, so that the patient really understands how important you consider oral hygiene to be.

Few devices

In principle, the patient should be instructed in the use of as few tooth-cleaning devices as possible. The larger the number of devices, the larger the risk that adequate tooth cleaning will not be performed. It is also important, that the devices you recommend, and supply the patient with in your office, are easily available at the pharmacy or elsewhere outside your office. If the patient cannot find the devices he was taught to use in a near-by store, established routines may break down, and your treatment may fail. It is also important that the patient understands how, and why, a particular device for interproximal cleaning e.g. tooth pick, or interproximal brush is used. Whenever possible the periodontal patient should use a proxa-brush. Flossing is not the procedure of choice in such patients.

It is nearly impossible to provide or describe in detail how a motivation and instruction procedure should be performed. Because you, the practitioner knows everything about the disease, its etiology and treatment, use your knowledge, imagination and dedication to transfer the message to the patient. Use the patient's language, and remember that your message should be based on knowledge rather than being technically oriented. If patients understand, they will adopt the cleaning procedure as their own and not something that was pushed on them. Be flexible, creative and individualize your talk and your behavior. The overall purpose is to establish a controlled procedure that should be evoked by or within the individual patient's inner self. Perhaps, you find this discussion superfluous or too simple. Do not forget though, that despite knowing about the need for interproximal cleaning for years, too many patients have been instructed to use toothpicks for *gingival massage* or *stimulation*, and not a single word has been uttered about the cleaning effect.

Sometimes you see patients using toothpicks for interproximal tooth cleaning in approximal spaces so large that it clearly reveals that the information has been totally misinterpreted. So again use your *imagination* to *individualize* your message, and make sure you receive *feedback* to ascertain that the patient has received your message correctly.

About motivation

1. **Create a good environment or atmosphere, and get to know your patient**
2. **Inform the patient about the disease**
3. **Make the patient aware that he/she has the (periodontal) disease**
4. **Inform the patient of possible consequences of the disease**
5. **Inform the patient of modulating and aggravating factors**
6. **Inform the patient about basic treatment and the specific treatment plan**
7. **Inform the patient about the importance of compliance**

About instruction

1. **Understand your patient's needs, knowledge and prejudices**
2. **Show the patient tooth and gum anatomy and their relationships**
3. **Show what areas need to be cleaned**
4. **Explain techniques, but do not be too authoritarian. Make the patient believe that he/she decides how to clean**
5. **Individualize the technique and devices according to the patient's needs**
6. **Be creative, use your imagination**

Important statements

1. Never say: a patient has a bad hygiene. (how would you react to that?)
   Say: You have this disease and to prevent it from coming back you must be better than everybody else in brushing your teeth.

2. Say: I can help you to stop this infection. But you must prevent it from coming back by brushing your teeth thoroughly.

3. Never say: this is a transmittable disease.
   Say: You have inhereted these bacteria from your parents, or in a family most members share a lot of bacteria. Some may be good for you – some may not.

CHAPTER 3

Mechanical Treatment –
A Matter of Systematics and Individualization

The *mechanical debridement* i.e. *scaling and root planing* together with motivation and instruction in oral hygiene, constitute the basis for a cause-related treatment of periodontal diseases. Sometimes this is called 'initial therapy' as if more therapy was inevitable. In fact, if well performed, *non-surgical periodontal therapy* would be sufficient in the majority of cases. It is not meaningful, however, to initiate a difficult, time-consuming mechanical treatment until the patient has adopted and proved to be able to maintain proper oral hygiene. Not until then, can a lasting effect of the debridement be expected. Sometimes though, the prerequisite for good oral hygiene has to be created by initial removal of supra-gingival calculus and restoration overhangs.

It must, therefore, be stressed *that the dentist or the dental hygienist has to put straightforward oral hygiene demands on the patient, and ensure that these are satisfied.*

If these demands are understood and accepted by the patient, the therapist can be strict in the evaluation, and delay further treatment until oral hygiene is acceptable. This may further contribute to the motivation of the patient, and make the patient realize the seriousness of the demands. Since the scaling and root planing procedures are usually done by the quadrant, every next appointment should begin with plaque control and the visualization of the plaque using a disclosing solution. This will further em-

phasize how important patient compliance is considered to be.

The mechanical debridement is a nonspecific treatment aiming at removing bacterial plaque (biofilm) and calculus from the root surfaces. By the scaling and root planing procedures bacteria, calculus and necrotic root cementum are removed in order to obtain the expected treatment results. At this point the *patient has the legal right to expect that this is accomplished, because this is what the patient is paying for.* Fig. 27a-f on p. 80 illustrates treatment outcome in a patient, in whom good oral hygiene and meticulous scaling and root planing resulted in resolution of the gingival inflammation, the establishment of healthy gingival tissue and a reduction of the periodontal pockets.

High quality scaling and root planing procedures are difficult and time consuming. Not every general practitioner is sufficiently involved or interested in periodontal therapy. However, if sufficient skill, time and dedication to properly perform periodontal treatment are absent, the patient will be at risk for further disease progression. Eventually, teeth may be lost and will have to be replaced with fixed or removable prosthetic appliances. Such outcomes cannot be considered satisfactory, in cases where properly performed periodontal treatment could have 'saved' the teeth. So, practitioners who are aware of their lack of knowledge, skills and clinical experience in periodontal therapy should feel the responsibility to refer the patient to a periodontist, when necessary. As a general practitioner you are not obliged to treat periodontal disease, but *you are obliged to diagnose* the diseases, and if present to *refer the patient* for treatment.

There may be several reasons why periodontal diagnosis, treatment and prevention are not routinely and adequately performed. One important reason, although no excuse, is that this element of dental care is often less profitable than restorative or prosthetic dentistry.

SYSTEMATIC MECHANICAL TREATMENT

Scaling and root planing

Having removed supragingival calculus and restoration overhangs, it is time for subgingival scaling and root planing. This part of the treatment aims at removing, plaque, calculus, tissue debris and toxic deposits, leading to the creation of a clean smooth root surface. Usually this implies that some cementum and dentin are removed. When present, root surface caries lesions should be dealt with.

Time consumption

One important prerequisite for success is that sufficient time is set aside to perform the treatment in an optimal way. A proper scaling and root planing procedure requires 25–45 minutes per quadrant for a skilled operator if the pockets are in the 4–5mm range. If the pockets are deeper, the procedure becomes significantly more difficult and more time is needed. Scaling and root planing procedures should be made without time pressure; without such stress, the patient will also

feel less pain and discomfort. Too vigorous use of instrumentation can tear open the pocket and create wounds that will cause pain. Because sub-gingival *scaling and root planing are time consuming and cause pain they should be performed under local anesthesia.*

Instrumentation

Selection of instruments – scalers and curettes – and the instrumentation itself, is dependent on the position of the tooth, the tooth/root anatomy, and the morphology of the periodontal defect. In addition, there are practical considerations such as working position to secure access to the defect. It is often preferable to sit in front of a patient who is sitting in a half-upright position, rather than behind a supine patient. The working position should be adjusted to the area in the oral cavity to be treated (Fig. 14).

Instruments

Machine instruments

Machine instruments as well as *hand instruments* are used for scaling and root planing. Modern non-surgical debridement should be based on the use of fine-tipped *ultrasonic scalers* or *sonic scalers*, and the additional use of hand instruments. Since the effect of ultra sonic and sonic scalers is based on oscillating movements, and since the removal of tooth substance can be considerable if these instruments are improperly used, it is of great importance to know the working concept of each specific instrument. In principle, the tip of ultra sonic (and sonic) instruments should be working along (parallel to) the root surface (Fig. 15a) and not against it. The latter will cause unnecessary damage to the root. Machine instruments are effective and ergonomically superior to hand instruments.

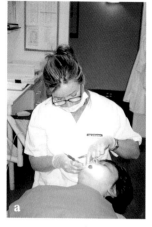
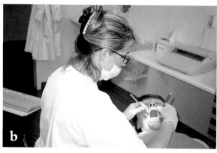
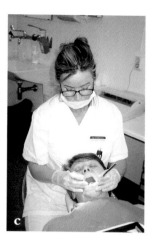

Fig 14 a - c Correct positioning when scaling and root planning in
a) side segments of upper jaws
b) side segments of lower jaws
c) front segment of upper and lower jaw.

Strength and energy can be saved, but *not time*. Rotating instruments such as the Waerhaug diamond (Fig. 15b) may occasionally be used in furcation areas and in root furrows and concavities, but should be used with great care. Machine instrumentation should always be supplemented with root planing by hand instrumentation in order to achieve a smooth root surface. Hand instruments

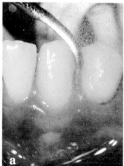
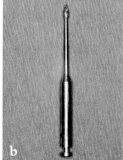

Fig 15 a,b
a) primary scaling using ultrasonic scaler
b) Waerhaugs diamond for rotating instruments.

provide better tactility to identify remaining irregularities and calculus on the root surface, and does less easily destroy the remaining periodontal ligament.

Hand instruments

In choosing hand instruments, They should be easy to grip and must not have a tendency to slip out of the operator's hand, otherwise unnecessary force must be used to hold it. The instruments should be designed to allow access to every root surface of the mouth. Also, the working parts should stay sharp during the entire scaling procedure.

Since the anatomy of teeth varies significantly between different tooth types and areas of the mouth, a great number of hand instruments are potentially needed to reach all areas. A well designed and well-maintained set of hand instrument should be regarded not only as a practical but also a cost effective investment for the clinic. Using too many instruments is too time consuming,

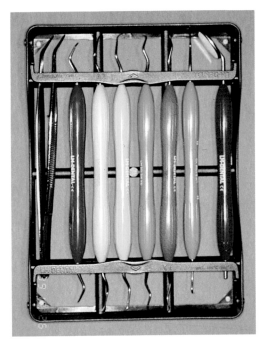

Fig 16 Our favourite cassette (the Preus-cassette) which should suffice in contents for the needs during regular scaling and root planing; periodontal probe, tweezers, mirror, Gracey curettes 11/22 mesial, Gracey curettes 13/14 distal, Colombia 2L/2R, Minisyntettes 215/216, Mini scalers LM23. (LM instruments OY, Finland)

since every change of instruments will constitute a break in the procedure. Every instrument is special, and demands a particular technique in order to achieve the proper angulation between the cutting edge and the root surface. Fig.16 shows a cassette of instruments put together by the authors. It contains:

Mirror
Periodontal probe
Gracey curette 11/12 mesial
Gracey curette 13/14 distal
Columbia 2L/2R
Mini syntette 215/216
Mini scaler LM 23
Tweezers

An additional cassette containing special instruments may occasionally be required. Diamond strips and rotating diamonds are included as well as special instruments for the removal of restoration overhangs such as: Harland's instrument, special knives, the Eva-system, and Profin Directional System with a special hand piece, and oscillating diamond tips. Even if these instruments are infrequently used, they are extremely valuable when needed.

Composite restorations are gradually increasing also in posterior areas. Too often these restorations have overhangs, which may be difficult to see. Such overhangs too frequently create local periodontal breakdown. Due to their plaque retention abilities, they have to be removed. Such removal is part of the scaling procedure, and can preferably be accomplished by the use of rotating or oscillating diamond tips.

Working with hand instruments, the curette is carefully moved down to the bottom of the pocket. The instrument is pressed against the tooth with the correct cutting edge angulation, and then moved in coronal direction along the root, or some times perpendicular to the root (Fig. 17). The curette should never be forced in apical direction, since this could cause tissue damage and constitute a risk for forcing bacteria into the tissue, with the possibility of a subsequent formation of an acute periodontal abscess. The movements are continuously repeated until the root surfaces are considered clean, as evaluated by tactile sounding of the root surface with a probe. By working *systematically,* no part of the root will be overlooked. Surface by surface, tooth by tooth. It is important always to have finger support when using hand instrumentation, partly to optimize precision in the movements, and partly to avoid finger cramps.

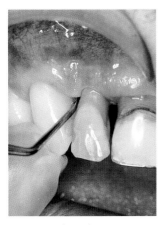

Fig 17 Scaling does not necessarily be performed in the axial direction of the tooth. Sometimes it may be convenient to scale in the circumferential direction too.

The instrument may not always be moved parallel to the tooth. Often it is more effective to move the curette along the root circumference, perpendicular to the long axis of the root. (Fig. 17) Both movements should be used. Reaching the bottom of the pocket with a curette or a sickle scaler the 'conventional way' is sometimes difficult but could be facilitated by reaching down with the tip of the curette, and moving it perpendicular to the root. The selection of instrument is always dependent on the anatomy of the periodontal defect. In narrow defects a mini-curette of appropriate design is recommended.

Sharpening of hand instruments

Sharpening of instruments should be performed between every treatment procedure in order to always have sharp instruments that effectively remove plaque and calculus and smoothens the root surface. Sharpening is done either by the use of a stone e.g. the Arkansas stone or the India stone, or a sharpening machine. Apart from getting a sharp edge sharpening also aims at restoring the correct working edge angle. An indicator of the instrument getting blunt is that more force is needed, and that the scaling movements are not smooth. If the instrument is slowly turned against the light a blunt cutting edge will reflect light, and appear as a light line. This is a sign that sharpening is required.

A sharpening stone is a less expensive alternative. However, in the hands of an untrained operator this is more difficult to use than a sharpening machine.

Some practitioners routinely sharpen their instruments during the treatment. Although sometimes necessary, it is not recommended. Sharpening the instrument in front of patients may look somewhat crude, and even stressing in particular by patients who have a certain degree of dental fear. Normally, if properly sharpened in advance, instruments should not have to be sharpened *during* the treatment procedure. Should the instrument become dull, which may happen during a long, full mouth scaling procedure, it is better to select a new and sharp curette instead of sharpening it during the procedure. Sharp instruments save time. It is therefore, recommendable to train the clinic staff, and to make one particular assistant responsible for this task.

Instruments may not only lose sharpness during treatment, but also during sterilization and storing. To minimize this, hand instrument are preferably sterilized and stored in a cassette. One example is the type shown in (Fig. 16) from LM instruments. To avoid instruments being thrown against each other the cassette should be designed to allow for separation of each instrument. An open cassette is recommended. Most manufacturer have these cassettes and none is preferable over the other.

The outcome of scaling and root planing depends on a series of factors such as: time allowed for each treatment procedure, selection and handling of instruments, working position, systematization on individual demands. The best outcome is achieved when all these factors are optimized.

PERIODONTAL SURGERY

Indications

Periodontal surgery may be performed after evaluation of the non-surgical treatment if:
Desired goals are not reached
Pockets continue to show signs of pathology and risk for disease progression.

Surgery as part of periodontal therapy is performed mainly for three reasons:
1. To create access for proper scaling and root planing in areas where closed debridement has failed or initially considered difficult to perform/likely to fail
2. To eliminate or reduce pocket depth, and
3. To regenerate periodontal tissues lost through the disease.

This part of the chapter will deal with indications for periodontal surgery in cases where pathological periodontal pockets remain after the non-surgical phase of therapy or in cases where a non-surgical approach primarily is considered insufficient for obtaining the goal of disease elimination.
It is impossible to provide standardized rules for when, and when not to perform surgery. Indications may vary from clinician to clinician, from patient to patient and between different areas and sites in the mouth. For example, one practitioner may successfully treat 7mm pockets without surgery, while another may require surgery to manage 5mm pockets. It is easier to scale a 7mm pocket mesial to a lateral incisor than distal to a low-er second molar. The decision has to be made by the practitioner who knows where to set his personal limit for success. If you feel that an area cannot be successfully treated non-surgically, it is an indication for surgery. But remember, *if you do not know how to perform scaling and root planing, surgery will not help.*

So before initiating periodontal therapy, the patient's situation and different treatment alternatives and treatment steps should be presented to the patient so that he or she can follow and understand the progress.

Surgery

A good discipline is to reserve surgical sessions to one clinic day per week. That will make the whole staff prepared for this task, and the procedures will run smoothly without unnecessary disturbances or interruptions. The operator and the assistants can focus on preparing for the procedures, to make sure that necessary equipment is available, all of which is important to minimize the risk for complications.

Do not plan for more than two surgical sessions during the morning, and two in the afternoon in the beginning. To minimize wound exposure, the time for a surgical procedure should nor exceed an hour and a half. The risks for post-surgical pain and infections increase with the time the wound is open. Therefore, the extension of the surgical field should be adjusted to the time factor and not because a patient wants it done in a hurry. The patient may have a long distance to travel and/or is very busy, and therefore would like to have as much done at every appointment as possible. In such situations the patient should be made aware of the risks and asked to compromise towards what is feasible, and what is best in terms of outcome of a successful surgical treatment.
Surgical procedures require special alertness

on the part of the operator that limits the time for the surgery to maintain high skill and quality. A better job is likely done if the surgical field is limited to a sextant or at the most a quadrant. If the surgery is extended the sharpness of mind, and the carefulness may fade, and the surgery may not be as successful as it should be. The result may even be worse than no surgery at all.

The patient's post-surgical comfort should not be forgotten or neglected. With surgeries performed on both sides in one sitting, eating may be difficult and healing compromised.

If scaling are to be performed the instrument kit should be carefully selected, and preferably limited to a few instruments. It is an advantage to have the instruments on a pre-prepared tray.

A minimum kit should include:
- mouth mirrors
- periodontal probe
- straight explorer
- cotton pliers
- tissue pliers
- scalpel handles for blades #12 and #15
- flap elevator according to Norberg or Hu-Friedy
- tissue scissors
- suture scissors
- curettes Hue Friedy 6/7 and 16/17 or Sandviken Y4 and Y5 mainly to remove granulation tissue
- Gracey or Mecca curettes selected according to experience including mesial and distal for scaling and root planing
- cassette with round burrs #1, 3, 5, 8 and flame-shaped diamond stone
- hemostat
- needle holder, preferably Castroviero
- sterile angulated hand piece
- spatula

In addition, the following is necessary:
- sterile disposable suction

- sterile (paper) cloths to cover patient, tray table, etc.
- sterile covers for drill tubes, etc.
- sterile surgical gloves preferably latex and powder free
- big sterile stainless bowl for saline solution
- big syringe and canula for saline irrigation

The disposable suction tube is adapted to the suction system of the unit. Repeatedly rinse the tube with saline. Always keep the wound humid through irrigation with saline. This will prevent post-surgical pain and promote healing. Repeated irrigation also keeps the surgical field clean and bright.

Important extra equipment such as a view-box for radiographs, holder for patient records with probing depths should also be mounted close to the operating table so that radiographs and probing data records can be easily looked at without having to leave the area.

Before the surgery is initiated the patient's medical history should be up-dated and medications checked to minimize risks for unexpected side effects and post-surgical complications. Remember; today patients visit their physician more frequently than before, and the patient may have gotten a new prescription from the doctor since the last appointment with you. At the same time the patient's previous medical status is confirmed or possible changes in general status and medication are established. Such extra check-ups will increase the patient's faith in the operator.

Surgical techniques

Flap procedure or gingivectomy? Is a question repeated over and over again? The gingivectomy is usually less complicated to perform than a flap procedure. However, these two procedures have different indications. Whatever procedure is chosen, it has to be performed with *minimum of trauma to the tissues*.

Indications for gingivectomy

The indications for gingivectomy are quite limited. Since the procedure implies that most of the supracrestal gingiva is excised. The depth of the gingival pocket should not exceed the width of gingiva propria. There are also esthetic concerns, since the procedure will result in significantly 'longer teeth'. The resultant root exposure leads to increased hypersensitivity against cold and heat. Furthermore, there must not be infrabony defects. So, consequently the only clear indication for gingivectomy is gingival enlargement or hyperplasia. However, the gingivectomy can be performed together with the flap procedure as for instance in the maxillary premolar, molar areas where a flap might be raised buccally, and the gingivectomy is performed in the palatal area.

Indications for flap procedures

1. Remaining periodontal pockets >5mm with bleeding on probing. The procedure is used as an access flap in order to perform open debridement, scaling and root planing. It is an 'open – clean – and close' procedure. Esthetics are mostly retained since the flap can be repositioned in its original position and secures good esthetic outcome.
2. Infrabony defects. Apart from providing access, the procedure is often combined with:
   • osteoplasty or osseous surgery for pocket elimination. This is usually accompanied by an apically repositioned flap resulting in somewhat longer teeth
   • regenerative procedures (See Chapter 5).

Periodontal surgery should in general be performed by a periodontist. For the general practitioner with special interest in periodontology it is still advisable to limit the surgical procedures to fairly simple cases. This can be compared with playing the piano; practicing a few times a month is not sufficient to maintain or gain skills.

The first phase of the surgery is anesthesia. This may be a stressful event for the patient. Always prepare the syringe out of sight of the patient, preferably in advance and placed on the surgery tray which is placed behind the patient. A careful, slow injection minimizes the pain to the patient. Remember, 'the needle' is what worries and stresses the patient most in advance. Therefore, anesthesia cannot be given too carefully, and might be initiated with topical anesthesia.

Gingivectomy

To guide the incision line buccal and lingual bleeding points (Figs. 18 a, b) are made at a level slightly apical to the bottom of the corresponding periodontal pocket. The scalpel is then brought through these bleeding points with a slight apical inclination of the incisions (Fig. 18 c). After completion of the incision the excised gingiva is removed (Fig. 18 d) and the wound area carefully inspected. If the incision is not deep enough and needs to be corrected at certain areas, the adjustment should start at the center of this area. Complete revision is difficult if the incision is started at the periphery. All granulation tissue and epithelium coronal to the incision line is removed. The exposed root surfaces are scaled and planed until they are clean and smooth (Fig. 18 e), and the surgical dressing, usually CEO PAC, is applied (Figs. 18 fg). The purpose is to cover and protect the wound surface during initial healing, and to minimize patient discomfort dur-

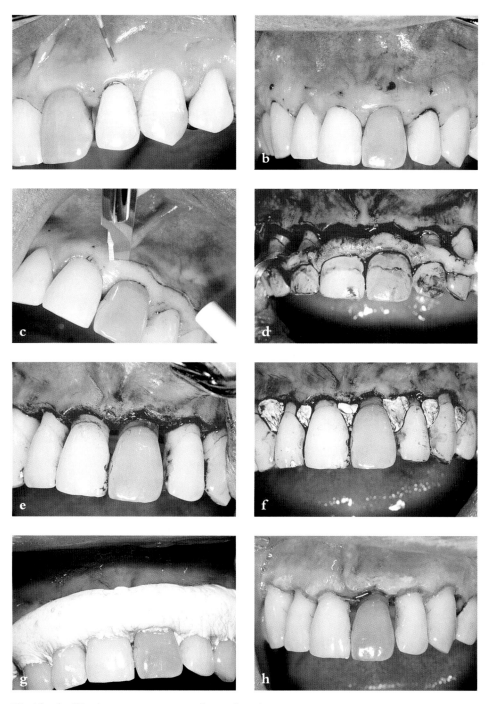

Fig 18 a-h Gingivectomy – see text for explanation.

ing the first post-surgical weeks. The dressing should cover the wound without interfering with the lip muscle activities, which may dislodge the dressing or create decubital wounds. The dressing is carefully packed interproximally in order to cover the interproximal wound surfaces, and to secure retention of the dressing (Fig. 18 f). The dressing is usually removed after 7–14 days (Fig. 18 h), which is the time needed for the new epithelium to cover the wound surface.

Modern periodontal flap procedures are basically performed in either of two ways:
– As a Modified Widman Flap procedure (MWF)
– As an Apically Positioned Flap procedure (APF)

While the MWF procedure mainly aims at creating access for open debridement, scaling and root planing, the APF is usually combined with some osseous plasty, osseous resection or osseous recontouring. The initial incisions are usually identical

Incision

The marginal incision can either be performed as an intra-sulcular incision or as a reversed bevel incision by which the gingiva margin and the inside of the gingival facing the root are excised. The reversed bevel incision is usually limited to the palatal aspect of the maxilla and preferably used when infrabony defects are present or when some kind of gingivoplasty is contemplated. The flap incisions are best extended one tooth mesial and distal to the target area. Make sure that the incision goes through the periosteum to the bone, otherwise the flap will be difficult to rise. The incisions should also go deep interproximally, in order to maintain as much of the papilla as possible. When possible, and in order to work non-traumatical-

ly without having to tear the tissues to achieve access, an oblique vertical release incision is made (Fig. 19 b) at the mesial extension of the flap. This mesial incision is made with the purpose of alleviation and for reducing the blood supply and nutrition to the flap during healing. An alternative to this procedure is to extend the incision one tooth further without including the papilla, which should be left untouched.

Flap elevation

Buccal and palatal mucoperiostal (full thickness) flaps are carefully raised, preferably using a Norberg or a Hu-Friedy elevator (Fig. 19c). The flap is raised just as much as needed to achieve good visibility of, and access to the target area. Be careful not to hurt the papilla!

Too much resistance in the flap is usually due to the fact that the incision has not completely penetrated the periosteum, or that the papilla has not been detached from the underlying granulation tissue.

Defect debridement and root surface instrumentation

Granulation tissue in intrabony defects is removed using curettes. Recommendable curettes are Sandviken Y4/Y5 or Hue Friedy 6/7 and 16/17. As the granulation tissue is rich in blood vessels profound bleeding often occurs before its removal. Scaling and root planing (S&RP) are performed much in the same manners as in closed S&RP procedures (Fig. 19 d). The inside of the flap is also curetted, in order to remove attached granulation tissue. This is accomplished with sharp scalpel blades, or with sharp tissue scissors (Fig. 19 e).

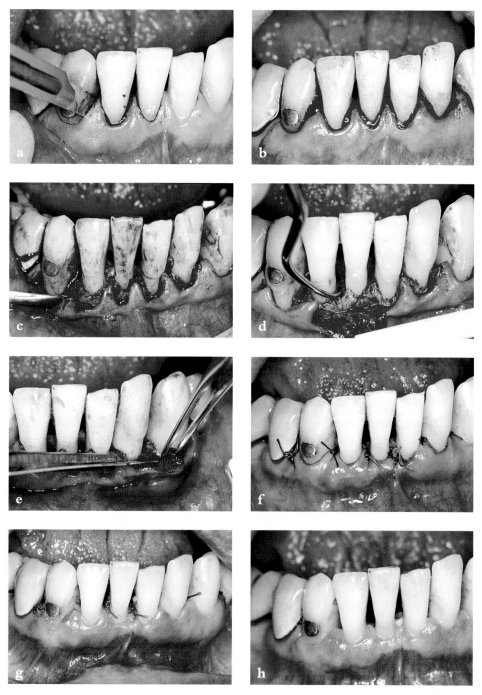

Fig 19 a – h Flap surgery – see text for explanation.

Bone resection

It is sometimes desirable to eliminate or reduce the depth of infrabony defects in order to accomplish pocket elimination. This is especially the case in multiple, moderately deep bony defects <4mm. Bony walls adjacent to bone defects are usually not supporting bone, so removing such bone does not impair the support to the tooth. For deeper defects periodontal regeneration procedures should be considered. Bone resection or bone plasty aiming at restoration of the bone anatomy are performed with rotating chisel burrs using great care and saline irrigation. Bone resection may occasionally include the removal of some bone supporting neighboring tooth/teeth. However, most often in such situation these neighboring teeth have optimal bone support, and will hardly suffer by losing a small amount of bone.

Suturing

Flap procedures are completed by repositioning and suturing of the flaps using usually single, interrupted sutures (Fig. 19f). Occasionally, continuous sutures are used. In case of the MWF procedure, the flaps are repositioned more or less in their original position. Following pocket elimination with osseous resection, the flaps are adjusted to the recontoured bone and sutured in a more apical position.

In both cases it is desirable to cover the interproximal bony crest, which is possible if the papillae have been preserved during incision and flap elevation. If not the flaps should be trimmed so as to elongate the papillae somewhat. The flaps are then *sutured together,* with no tension in the flap. The wound edges of the flaps should be related and then just held together with the suture. It is not possible to successfully force a flap in position or to bring the papillae together

with the suture. In most cases it is sufficient with one suture in each interproximal area. When sealing the releasing incision one may need 2–3 sutures to cover the exposed bone.

It cannot be emphasized enough that sutures are used to secure the wound edges to each other, and that there should be no tension in the flap when the suturing is finished. To accomplish tension-free suturing it is sometimes advantageous to make a horizontal releasing incision through the periosteum at the base of the flap. This will significantly increase the mobility of the flap and increase its management. The flaps will shrink somewhat, both during the surgery and during the initial post-surgical healing. Where there is initial tension, the sutures will cut through the tissue, and result in tissue ruptures, gingival recessions and/or interproximal soft tissue craters.

When choosing between straight or curved suture needles, it should be taken into consideration that curved needles have a force vector acting in the radius of the needle with a tendency to traumatically cut the tissue. This will not happen with a straight needle. The authors prefer using straight needles.

The use of a surgical pack or dressing may be indicated following an APF flap procedure and may help to keep the flap in position. Normally the use of a pack is not necessary following a flap procedure, and especially if the soft tissues have been preserved and complete soft tissue coverage of the underlying bone is envisaged.

Sutures are removed after 10–14 days (Figs. 19 g, h). Also, if a surgical pack was used, it is left in place until the time of suture removal.

Post-surgical complications

Post-surgical complications do occur. However, with careful surgery techniques they are limited to a minimum. If complications still occur, it is important to be able to understand why, and to be able to respond.

Edema occurs now and then and is usually most apparent following the second day, after which it gradually disappears. The reason is mainly that the circulatory systems for blood and lymph are severed during the surgery, resulting in leakage of blood and lymph into the subcutaneous tissues. It takes a while until the shunts are closed, and normal rheology is re-instituted. Therefore, the patient should be informed about the risk of swelling, but also that it will soon disappear. Chilling over the treated area directly with ice after surgery for about 30 minutes may significantly prevent the development of edema. If edema has occurred, a warm pack over the area may accelerate its resorption.

The use of antiphlogistics may also prevent edema. However, *make sure the patient is not sensitive/allergic to the drug.*

Edema increases tension to the sutures with increased risk for the sutures to cut through the tissues that then may disrupt and even recede. As this, in turn, may result in partial or complete failure, all precautions should be undertaken to avoid complications. If the flaps have been properly repositioned and sutured without tension, there is a safety margin to compensate for the swelling. Yet, it is important to notice early signs of edema and try to counteract the effects.

Pain is relatively frequent following gingivectomy due to the large wound surface area, but less frequent following flap procedures. Pain due to the trauma usually appears shortly after surgery. It is therefore recommended to give the patient some kind of painkiller immediately after the surgery, (before the local anesthesia has been metabolized) and to continue the medication throughout the first 24 hours. Pain increas-

es the release of prostaglandins and healing will be delayed. Sustained or extended pain may occur in cases of over-long surgery with extended bone exposure, drying out of the wound area during excessive suction, and over-tight sutures. On the other hand, it is well to remember that great variations exist as to patients' pain thresholds.

Antiphlogistic drugs can, to some extent, prevent or reduce pain. Antiphlogistics like *ibuprofen* have both an analgesic and an antipyretic effect. Although very infrequent, pain may last for several days and can be very intense. In such cases, stronger painkillers including codeine are prescribed (Codeine is a drug that affects the opium receptors in the CNS). However, *be sure that the pain is not caused by infection that is masked by the use of strong analgesics.*

Post-surgical infections are infrequent, but do occur. Pain that appears some days after surgery is most likely due to infection of the wound. Post-surgical use of an antiseptic mouth rinse, such as a Chlorhexidine solution, usually prevents the infection. If the patient develops fever and general malaise, antibiotic therapy should be started. Ordinary penicillin 1g bid. is usually sufficient. For those who are allergic to penicillin, equivalent doses of chlindamycin are recommended. Patients on antibiotics should be monitored to avoid the risk of specific bacteria being resistant to the antibiotic.

Loosened sutures are of no consequence if the wound has already healed. Often too many days have passed since the suture actually loosened, and there is no real purpose in the suture. The purpose of the suture is to keep the flaps in place, and if the suture has failed, it has to be replaced. In case of a minor tissue disruption interproximally, the tissue will re-form with time without further adjustment. If the flap has sloughed, resuturing may be necessary. Usually, however, the wound surfaces do re-epithelialize and it becomes necessary to create fresh wound surfaces that can be sutured to each other. If the soft tissue defect is too large, as with a negative papilla or interproximal soft tissue crater, some gingivoplasty is necessary. A negative papilla makes interproximal cleaning difficult and produces a risk for disease recurrence.

Post-surgical instruction and care

Post-surgical instruction is mandatory after every periodontal intervention:
- no mechanical tooth cleaning in the operated area for 2–4 weeks
- prophylactic analgesics for 24 hours
- twice daily rinsing with Chlorhexidine solution
- avoiding course food stuffs and excessive mastication.
- if problems occur call the surgeon.

All surgery should be well planned and executed with full consent of the patient The patient should also be well prepared at the time of surgery. Thus, post-surgical instructions are just repetition of previous conversations.

If essential post-surgical instructions are delivered for the first time to an exhausted and partially confused patient immediately following surgery, the likelihood is that the information will not be understood. This can easily be avoided if the patient is well informed in advance. There are, however, still reasons to supply patients with written, easy-to-understand information directly after the surgery that can be read in the comfort of their own home.

Mouth rinsing. The patient should be instructed not to eat or drink within 3 hours after surgery and to rinse the mouth with a 0.2% Chlorhexidine solution for 1 minute twice daily for 2–4 weeks, starting the day after surgery. The patient should be given the first bottle of the mouth rinse in the office, with the recommendation to purchase additional bottles in the pharmacy. Chlorhexidine attaches to the tooth and epithelial surfaces and prevents bacterial colonization and plaque formation and infection of the wound. Once the sutures have been removed, mouth rinsing can be substituted by local application of 1.0% Chlorhexidine gel.

Mechanical tooth cleaning (tooth brushing) should not be performed in the area of surgery during the first 2–4 weeks of healing. Plaque control in the area is accomplished by Chlorhexidine rinsing. Once mechanical tooth brushing is resumed, it should be initially supervised, and if necessary adjusted to possible anatomical changes produced by the operation, e.g. larger interproximal spaces may need larger interproximal brushes.

Antibiotics. While antibiotic therapy in conjunction with periodontal surgery is widely used in Southern Europe, USA and Latin America, it is used on very strict and defined indications in the Scandinavian countries. There are two possible indications:

1. General antibiotic prophylaxis for serious medical conditions. In such cases *3 g of Amoxicillin or equivalent doses of Clindamycin are given 1 hour prior to surgery. If allergic to penicillin, the regimen of choice would be 600mg Clindamycin 1 hour prior to surgery.*
2. Severely advanced periodontitis caused by specific pathogens (See Chapter 4).

Recently this regimen has been challenged since it seems more die from anaphylaxia than endocarditis. However, one should stick with this regimen as long as authorities do not change them officially.

Prophylactic antibiotics as a complement to periodontal surgery are used only occasionally, and then based on microbiological tests and evaluation of antibiotic resistance.

Analgesics and antiphlogistics (e.g. Ibuprofen 600mg post-surgically is recommended for the first 24–48 hours). Apart from preventing/relieving pain these compounds also reduce the risk for post-surgical edema. *Be sure the patient is not sensitive to ASA,* in which cases other types of painkillers e.g. paracetamol, are used. If the patient experiences pain 3–4 days after surgery, infection should be suspected, and the patient should see the dentist for examination and diagnosis. What treatment is then given will depend on the reason for the pain. As painkillers we specifically recommend 400 mg ibuprofen combined with 500 mg paracetamol every 4–5 hours until pain is tolerable or gone, thus targeting the inflammatory as well as the neurologically derived pain. Normally, there is no need for further medication after the first few hours.

Staining. The teeth, white restorations, and the tongue may develop a brown–grey stain in conjunction with the Chlorhexidine rinsing. (The stain is not due to the Chlorhexidine per se, but to pigments in coffee, tea, wine, herbs etc. which are attached to the Chlorhexidine treated tissue surfaces.) This is something the patient should be informed about in advance. Stain on the teeth is removed by professional polishing with polishing pastes. Stain on the tongue disappears after the rinsing is withdrawn. The patients often experience these stains as sign of disease. Therefore, it is important to show the patient that we care, by regularly and intermittently removing the stain. This also increases the patient motivation to complete the rinsing, which is so important for a good healing and treatment outcome.

Further information. Patients should be informed about the most common post-surgical events and possible complications and

their symptoms in order to know when to call the clinic. Pain more than 1–2 days post-surgically should not occur. Surgical dressings, when used can come loose and sutures do disrupt sometimes. If that occurs late in the healing period, no replacements are necessary.

A little extra concern pays. Nobody likes to be operated upon. That is why it is so important to give the patient a little extra attention. Small talk and expressions of empathy prior to surgery may serve to relax the patient. Calm and confident behavior is reassuring. Make sure the patient is brought in on time. Extended waiting can cause anxiety and be painful in particular before a surgical experience. Light conversation with your assistant during the surgery, especially about something interesting will distract the patient. Following completion of the surgery, talk to the patient; give your home telephone number at which you can be reached in the evening (do not be afraid, calls rarely materialize). And, do not to forget to call the patient in the evening or the day after, to make sure everything is all right. This will not only give you a loyal, appreciating patient, you will also learn how very seldom complications occur.

Post-surgical follow-up

Sutures and surgical dressing are removed 10–14 days after surgery. It is often advantageous to maintain the sutures for an extended period to minimize the risk for flap retraction. The patient should preferably still be seen a week after surgery. A prerequisite to keep the sutures for another week is that they are still in place and do not cause irritation to the wound area.

Chlorhexidine rinsings should be continued until the patient can resume mechanical tooth cleaning. However, interproximal cleaning can be augmented by dipping the Proxa Brush in Chlorhexidine solution or gel.

Once a surgical dressing is removed, e.g. after a gingivectomy, the wound surface is covered with a whitish layer consisting of exfoliated epithelium. This epithelium is easily, but carefully washed off with a gauss soaked with saline. Remember that the wound surface may still be tender and sore.

Soft tissue healing after flap surgery is fairly well completed after 2–4 weeks, providing that the sutures effectively supported the flap. Pain or soreness is infrequent if complications have not occurred.

Occasionally interproximal healing results in a negative papilla. Such an interproximal concavity may constitute a plaque trap, and should be adjusted.

There are several possible reasons for the development of a negative papilla:

- Too much interproximal tissue was removed during the incision without subsequently trimming, reshaping and coronally advancing the flap before suturing
- Sutures have opened or torn off
- Sutures have been too tight and cut through the flap tissue
- The papillae may have been thinned too much resulting in impairment of blood supply and nutrition to the tissue and necrosis of the papillae .

A negative papilla impairs the possibilities for cleanliness in the area. However, if not too deep, these soft tissue craters will reform with time. If remodeling does not occur, a gingivoplasty may be performed. Such interventions can usually be performed with an eletrotome.

Supportive care
Once the patient has resumed mechanical tooth cleaning (tooth-brushes and devices for interproximal cleaning) regular monitoring and supervision of plaque control is mandatory. Plaque control appointments and professional tooth cleaning based on individual needs, should be scheduled at least once every month during the first 6 months of healing. After 6 months the intervals of supportive care should be based on patients' needs, compliance and other factors of importance for disease recurrence.

Re-evaluation and long-term follow-up
Reevaluation of treatment outcome after surgery by probing depth and/or clinical attachment level measurements is not performed until 6 months after surgery, which is the time needed for tissue maturation and remodeling. Continuous follow-ups and supportive care are given according to disease severity and patients' needs in very much the same manner as following non-surgical therapy. Re-evaluation and supportive care is further discussed in *Chapter 6*.

CHAPTER 4

The Use of Antibiotics in Periodontal Disease Control

The most common and accepted treatment for periodontal diseases is conventional mechanical treatment. As shown in Chapter 3, conventional mechanical treatment produces a predictive, successful outcome if the patient is able to perform an adequate oral hygiene. What we actually do by performing a conventional mechanical therapy is to target a non-specific infection with a non-specific method, and to 'tidy up a complex infection'. Many clinical studies support the use of mechanical therapy in the treatment of periodontal diseases, but it is mostly the moderately to slowly progressing infections that respond to such therapy. Thus it is important to clearly acknowledge the individuality of the disease as well as the strengths and the limitations of the treatment modalities, and the high skills and adequate instruments that are required. There is a small group of periodontal sites and pockets that does not respond to mechanical therapy, or responds only partly. The reason for this may be

1. Inadequate mechanical treatment (including oral hygiene practices) or difficult anatomical configurations or other conditions
2. Specific infection, which is not curable by mechanical means alone, and
3. Re-infection from the surrounding structures (cheeks, tongue and other periodontalsites), or from other people with whom one is often in contact.

Re. 1 above. Dull instruments and inadequate techniques are the most common reasons for treatment failure. These are easily recognizable deficiencies, and should suggest to the practitioner that the patients should be referred to a specialist in periodontology. There is absolutely nothing wrong or embarrassing in the fact that a general practitioner dislikes or does not manage to treat periodontal diseases. However, it is wrong not to give his patients the option to be treated properly by specialists.

Re. 2 above. Specific infections are infections where one or several bacteria can be associated with the infection. Frequently these infections are not eliminated by mechanical treatment alone, especially since these organisms have certain pathogenic features which allow them to invade gingival tissues or to recolonize the pocket after treatment. It is also completely impossible to remove all bacteria from a periodontal pocket by mechanical means. The remaining flora with a high percentage of specific pathogenic bacteria, may then contribute to the recurrence of disease.

Re. 3 above. *Actinobacillus actinomycetemcomitans* and *Porphyromonas gingivalis* seem to colonize family members according to different transmission patterns. Generally, *A. actinomycetemcomitans* transmits from parents to children, but seldom/never between spouses. *P. gingivalis* seems to spread among all family members as soon as it enters a family, and the transmission is without specific routes. This opens the possibility that *P. gingivalis* may reinfect a family member recently treated for periodontal disease, if other family members are infected. Studies of transmission of other bacteria, (except *P. intermedia*), have not been performed, but it is likely that other periodontal pathogens may produce recurrent disease in the same manner. It is difficult to see how *A. actinomycetemcomitans* may cause frequent recurrent disease by transmission from exogenous donors. *A.actinomycetemcomitans* seldom/never transmits between spouses and does not easily colonize an already 'mature' microflora. However, transmission of *A.actinomycetemcomitans* is theoretically possible, since a microflora in reorganization after periodontal treatment may accept exogenous bacteria. Re-infection with *A. actinomycetemcomitans* may most probably be due to contamination from other areas in the oral cavity.

Antibiotic therapy

In some few cases, a well-performed mechanical treatment followed by an adequate oral home care program may not result in remission of disease. This may occur generally or just in certain periodontal sites. In such cases, the general practitioner must investigate if these cases are true periodontal diseases or could be other periodontal conditions such as those described in the section on differential diagnosis (in Chapter 1). If other conditions can be excluded, and the clinical condition is inconsistent with the criteria for a periodontal infection, one should start to think 'specific infection', and in this extended therapeutic concept, assess the possibility of using antibiotic or chemotherapeutic approaches in the treatment of this patient. Fig. 20 helps you to decide. There are clear guidelines for the adjunct treatment of periodontal diseases with antibiotics.

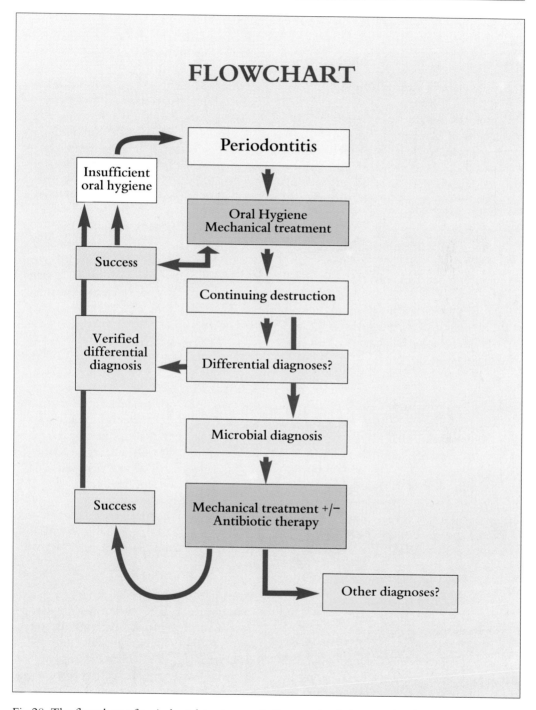

FLOWCHART

Periodontitis

Insufficient oral hygiene

Oral Hygiene Mechanical treatment

Success

Continuing destruction

Verified differential diagnosis

Differential diagnoses?

Microbial diagnosis

Success

Mechanical treatment +/− Antibiotic therapy

Other diagnoses?

Fig 20 The flowchart of periodontal treatment. A diagram that helps you decide which strategies to apply in different situations may come in handy when treating different periodontal diseases.

Adjunct antibiotics should be employed in the following scenarios:

Refractory periodontal disease

Periodontitis that does not respond to optimal mechanical treatment, and where most teeth continue to lose attachment despite meticulous mechanical treatment and a flawless oral hygiene, i.e. a periodontitis which has not received adequate treatment.

Advanced Periodontitis (Young, aggressive)
(Previously called „juvenile periodontitis")

Antibiotic therapy may be warranted already in the first phase of the treatment if the clinical and microbiological diagnosis coincides with this narrow diagnosis.

Rapidly Progressing Periodontitis

Periodontal disease that has been observed over some time, and where there has been at least 2mm attachment loss over a comparatively short period of time, despite a flawless oral hygiene. Since this diagnosis cannot be derived at without preceding mechanical treatment and observation time, one may institute the antibiotic therapy as soon as microbiological diagnosis confirms the tentative clinical diagnosis.

Acute Periodontal Abscess

If a patient shows fever, fatigue and general malaise antibiotic therapy should be administered as soon as possible. *The abscess must be incised, if possible through the pocket or the gingival mucosa.*

Rational for the use of antibiotics in periodontal disease control

- The disease to be treated must be a periodontal, bacterial infection
- The periodontal infection must be a specific infection.
- Target bacteria for the antibiotic treatment must be known
- An antibiotic must be available that targets the periodontal pocket (target area)
- Prophylactic use antibiotics
- The chosen antibiotic must give as few side effects as possible
- The chosen antibiotic must cause as little resistance development as possible

---

Differential diagnosis

As discussed in Chapter 1, the diagnosis of **specific periodontal infection** can be claimed only after a microbiologic test. A mixed flora, with no specific putative periodontal pathogens cannot be considered a specific infection. This may be a sign that the mechanical treatment has been a failure for other reasons than the presence of a specific infection, or that the bacterial test was wrong. This calls for referral to a specialist, and a new mechanical strategy including surgery.

If the microbiological test shows that specific periodontopathic microorganisms are present in high numbers, antibiotic treatment should be instituted. The number of pathogenic bacteria sufficient to produce disease varies from species to species depending on their virulence and pathogenic features, but as far as *A. actinomycetemcomitans* and *P.gingivalis* are concerned, it is estimated that a concentration of 100,000 cells or more per ml sample is pathognomonic. By performing a microbiological test, one gets to know which microorganisms will be the targets of the therapy. Thus it is of the essence to perform the mechanical treatment before even thinking about the possibilities of a specific infection. Without such strategy, the microbiological diagnosis will display, at best, a too complicated and at worst a totally wrong result. The treatment consists of a repeat of the mechanical treatment and an adjunct antibiotic therapy.

An antibiotic must target the periodontal pocket

Based on the microbiological test, the clinician has an array of antibiotics to choose from, but it is not desirable to select an antibiotic solely based on the test. The test is performed in a laboratory, and several clinical features are not taken into consideration. One important point is that the antibiotic must gain access to the periodontal pocket (target area). There is no use in selecting an antibiotic which has a high concentration in the kidneys or skin but relatively low concentration in the periodontal target area. The antibiotics of choice in periodontal disease control must be present in high concentrations in the gingival crevicular fluid (GCF).

Conventional penicillin is not predictably active in periodontal pockets due to the fact that 1/3 of all sub-gingival biofilms contain bacteria that produce penicillinases. Penicillinases are enzymes that destroy penicillin molecules, rendering them useless to fight infection.

Another important thing is that the antibiotic, enters the pocket through the GCF *in a certain molecular configuration*. To produce an antimicrobial effect, the antibiotic molecule must associate and bind to the outer membrane of the bacterium. Antibiotic molecules are quite indiscriminative in their approach to bacteria, and both the pathogenic and the non-pathogenic microorganisms bind antibiotic molecules. The success of an antibiotic rests on the fact that there has to be a comparatively higher number of antibiotic molecules to the number of bacteria that bind the antibiotic. If there are too many bacteria (pathogenic and non-pathogenic) binding the antibiotic, there will be pathogenic bacteria present that are not destroyed after treatment, leaving a population of live target bacteria that after treatment may re-infect the target area, and produce recurrence of disease. Moreover a biofilm is inert to antibiotics by definition. Thus the structure of the biofilm needs to be disrupted in order to gain success from the antibiotic used. To prevent this from happening, it is of utmost importance to reduce the amount of bacteria , i.e. scaling and root planning, in the pocket prior to antibiotic treatment.

This scheduling of the antibiotic administration within the entire clinical treatment, depends on how many visits it takes to perform the mechanical therapy and the duration of the antibiotic regimen. One cannot trust the previously performed scaling, because it is at least 3 months old. This is another reason for always performing a very thorough initial mechanical therapy, and thus one may spend less time and effort in the repeated procedure. If 2 visits are needed to perform the mechanical treatment, the antibiotic therapy may start on the day of the first visit if there is less than a week in between. If 3 or more sessions are needed, the antibiotic treatment may start between the penultimate and last visit. A 3-week antibiotic treatment will cover most mechanical treatments completely, and should not give too many problems. Most modern antibiotic treatments should last for 7–14 days. However, when tetracyclines are used (although rare) against *A. actinomycetemcomitans* 3 weeks of treatment is desirable.

Antibiotic prophylaxis

Prophylactic use of antibiotics is indicated in patients with dysfunctional or transplanted heart valves, rheumatic fever or in all patients that have the potential to develop endocarditis. Some scholars maintain that such prophylactic treatment should be instituted in patients with any transplant/implant in his cardiovascular system. Others would provide prophylactic antibiotics only to patients with such transplants/implants close to the heart muscle itself.

Periodontal or restorative treatments that warrant such prophylactic antibiotics are those that may cause bleeding, i.e. scaling, subgingival filling therapy where bleeding may be provoked, as well as endodontic therapy.

Prophylactic treatment consist of either 2g or 3g Amoxicillin 1 hour before treatment. A recommended dosage of 3g has been deemed necessary to provide an effective cover. In USA the dosage was changed to 2g in 1997, and it is expected that within the not too distant future all countries will recommend a dosage of 2g instead of 3g. If the patient is allergic to penicillin, 600mg Clindamycine 1 hour before treatment is recommended instead.

Side effects of prophylactic antibiotic cover are almost non-existent since it involves one single dose. However, there is always the possibility for an allergic reaction towards penicillin.

As earlier stated this regimen is under scruteny, and may be recommended against in the future. However, for now we have to comply with this convention.

The risks for side effects must be minimal when selecting an antibiotic. Since we have so many antibiotics to choose from, the consideration of unwanted effects must be

taken into account in every single case. It is also important to perform a microbiological test before selecting an antibiotic.

Known side effects of systemic antibiotic therapy are gastro-intestinal problems, such as: nausea, vomiting, diarrhea and sharp stomachaches (specifically caused by intake of metronidazol). Some patients feel headaches, weakness and fatigue. When side effects like these are frequently experienced, it is important to look out for more serious sequelae. If the diarrhea becomes too frequent and the patient is losing to much liquid, or the side effects cannot be tolerated for the short period of time, the therapy should end. However, it is possible to alleviate most gastrointestinal side effects by eating yogurts 2–3 times per day. The antibiotics should be taken 30 min. before, or 2hrs after a meal. However, in case of stomachaches the antibiotic may be taking *with* the meal.

Two antibiotics, Amoxicillin and Clindamycine, may produce a severe condition called pseudomembranous colitis. This is caused by resistant *Clostridium difficile* and its toxins. This infection may cause a bloody and mucous diarrhea, which may seriously dehydrate the patient. Ending the antibiotic treatment will normally lead to recovery. However, sometimes intravenous fluid administration is needed, and in the worst cases one may have to administer specific antibiotics against *C. difficile*. Hospitalization may become necessary but ordinarily prognosis is good. Contact the patients physician if you feel that you do not master the situation.

Resistance development

As clinicians, with the right to prescribe antibiotics, we have taken on a great responsibility. As we have just seen, antibiotics may cause side effects. However, more important is the danger for resistance development, which inevitably follows the use of these drugs. This side effect will inevitably cause changes in the environment in a longer perspective, and thus we would urge the prescribers to be cautious and correct when prescribing them.

Since the commercialization of penicillin more than 60 years ago, the use of antibiotics has exploded. Antibiotics have been used to control infections, in fish, meat and dairy production, with careless, non-reflective attitudes, that have caused unwanted and unexpected results. Antibiotics are not predictably useful any more. Today hundreds of thousands people die every year from infections that cannot be treated by any known single, or combinations of, antibiotics. This has been an increasing problem, and will be for years to come, only prevented and slowed by a reduced, careful and competent use of these drugs.

In essence resistance is a way for microorganisms to avoid the effect of an antibiotic. This may happen as a result of mutation and selection of resistant organisms during a selective pressure from antibiotics. Or it may actually happen through transfer between bacteria of DNA sequences that code for resistance traits. Such transfer may be the result of transfer through sex-pili, bacteriophage activity or uptake of naked DNA from the environment.

Natural selection of resistant microorganisms always happens in the sub-gingival plaque when an antibiotic is used. Normally direct, recognizable effects are not observed by such changes, but in a longer perspective such changes may be detrimental to the environment. The development of periodontal periapical abscesses may result from such selective pressure. Such abscesses may be the result of the use of antibiotics for

other infections than those purely related to periodontal disease, e.g. vaginitis, sinusitis or others. Use of antibiotics in such cases may cause selection of specific bacteria in periodontal and dental foci, resulting in abscess formation. These abscess formations are less frequent when treating periodontal infections with antibiotics, since the antibiotic is only administered as an adjunct to mechanical therapy. Nevertheless, the question is: Should a physician obtain information about the periodontal/dental status of the patient before administering antibiotics for any reason? Our view on this is clear: The use of antibiotics – for any reason – should not be performed without prior assessment of oral infections.

As already pointed out, antibiotics may alter the nucleotide sequence in the DNA of human cells. Antibiotics of special interest in this connection are the Quinolones. This group of antibiotics is designed to target the bacterial topoisomerase (gyrase), an enzyme implicated in the 'packing' process of DNA after mitosis. Hypothetically, even if designed to target bacterial DNA, the antibiotic may also affect the human DNA. Importantly, this has not been shown.

Mutations may on its own produce resistance against antibiotics. For every 40,000 −100,000 generations there is a statistically possibility for mutation, and if this results in a biologically beneficial change in the bacterial ability to adjust to the present environment, this will provide for a new clone of bacteria. If a mutation occurs under the influence of an antibiotic, and this mutation results in increased ability to resist the antibiotic, a new clone of resistant bacteria is produced. Most commonly the new, resistant strain will be reduced or vanish completely when the antibiotic regimen is ended. Finally, there is the risk that the resistant strain will remain in the ecosystem, resulting in possible failure in use of antibiotics in later and more serious or fatal, incidences of infection.

The problems of bacterial resistance to antibiotic treatment are no longer solely a scientific issue, but a concern to public health. In 1994 Newsweek and Time magazines carried extensive articles on antibiotic resistance, which provided a pretty grim future for control of infections. Both learned and lay now agree that it is important to reduce the use of antibiotics, and that they should be prescribed only when necessary, and that a correct procedure be followed: tests, selection of the correct antibiotic, choosing the right regimen, and extensive follow-up.

The development of bacterial resistance against an antibiotic occurs because the microorganism has:
1. Changed its surface so that the antibiotic molecule cannot recognize its site of attachment
2. Developed an ability to release the antibiotic molecules out of the cell as soon as it has gained access
3. Changed the configuration of the target structure, and
4. Developed a way to inactivate the antibiotic molecule.

Whatever the reason, such antibiotic resistance may be transferred from one bacterial cell to the next. This is especially evident in bacteria where resistance genes are located in a plasmid, and not on the bacterial chromosome itself. Plasmids are small DNA 'rings' in the bacterial cytoplasm which commonly code for antibiotic resistance or other pathogenic features, and which readily may be transferred to other bacteria by several routes. They may transfer through sex-pili; they may be packed in bacterial vira called bacteriophages; or they may be transferred as naked DNA when taken up by living bacteria after being released into the environment following death and destruction of the bacterial cell. If a microorganism carries such plasmids, they may acquire resistance genes of various qualities and against several antibiotics and thereby become multiresistant. Plasmids, which code for multiresistance, may be transferred to other bacteria. This way it is not difficult to understand how antibiotic resistance may spread and pose a quickly growing problem to our society.

As one can see, there are many possibilities for microorganisms to achieve antibiotic resistance. It is also clear that this development occurs most often in closely packed bacteria, and under the proper temperature. Such conditions are most prominent in the intestines, but also – and perhaps more so – in supra- and sub-gingival bacterial biofilms. Therefore, dental practitioners carry an obvious responsibility to intellectualize these mechanisms, and to work to prevent resistance development, since the mouth contains a multiple micro-environment where such mechanisms exist.

Types of antibiotics and antiseptics in periodontal disease control

Tetracyclines find little use in the treatment of periodontal diseases, although normally they are used as an alternative antibiotic when treating *A. actinomycetemcomitans* infections. Tetracyclines should be used where other antibiotics cannot be used for different reasons, but it should be abundantly clear that tetracyclines are the antibiotics to which bacteria develop resistance fastest and most effectively. Tetracyclines are broad-spectered bacteriostatic compounds, i.e. they only inhibit growth of the targeted bacteria, not killing them.

Metronidazole is effective in treatment of periodontal diseases associated with anaerobic bacteria like *P. gingivalis* and *P. intermedia*. *A. actinomycetemcomitans* may also be affected through metabolites, although normally being resistant to this, narrow spectered bactericidal. Side effects are few.

Ciprofloxacine is mostly used when microbiologic tests have ascertained that a superinfection with bacteria like enterobacteria, pseudomonads or staphylococci is present. The antibiotic is a very broad spectered bactericidal drug, which should be used only in situations of specific diagnosis. Side effects are quite uncommon.

Chlorhexidine is not an antibiotic, this broad-spectered antiseptic has shown great efficacy in preventing and treating gingival inflammations. Both rinsing solutions and sub-gingivally prepared formulations can be used in both bacterial and fungal infections.

Combination therapy consisting of metronidazole and penicillin (i.e. Amoxicillin), or metronidazole and Ciprofloxacine, has proven effective against *A. actinomycetemcomitans* infections. The bactericidal and broad spectered combination is very powerful, but carries with it a high-frequency of side effects, including a very severe diarrhea.

Antifungal dugs. It is not infrequent to find fungi as part of the microflora in periodontitis, especially in asthma patients. Studies suggest that as much as 10–15% of periodontal diseases are associated with fungi of various types – especially Candida species. Fungus in periodontal diseases must be considered as superinfections, and should be managed properly before instituting specific antibacterial therapy, since the latter may enhance the fungal overgrowth by suppressing the bacteria. Nystatin and Flukonazol are potent fungicides.

Selection of antibiotics based on microbiological tests

Primary infection with *A. actinomycetemcomitans* alone, or in combination with other bacteria should be treated by combination therapy. Although this has not been formally accepted in medical and pharmaceutical textbooks, the following regimen is endorsed in the world literature: Metronidazole tablets: 750mg per day in combination with 1250mg Amoxicillin per day for 8 days. Side effects may be stomach pain and other gastrointestinal problems as well as a severe diarrhea due to pseudomembranous colitis. Amoxicillin may cause allergies. In case of allergy or other reasons for not using this combination therapy, one may administer tetracyclines for 3 weeks, or Ciprofloxacine for 10 days.

Primary infection with *P. gingivalis, P. intermedia, Fusobacterium spp* and other anaerobic bacteria calls for the use of Metronidazol alone. 1250–1500mg per day for 10 days. Metronidazole may cause sharp stomach aches, which can be prevented by taking the drug with the meals. Patients should be told that metronidazol and alcohol may sometimes act together to elicit an antabus effect, which is extremely uncomfortable.

Enterobacter, E. coli, pseudomonads, Shigella and other are the most commonly occurring super infections. The treatment consists of Ciprofloxacine 500mg x 2 per day in 10–14 days, or tetracyclines 100mg (low dose) or 1000mg (high dose) per day for 14 days, depending on the results of microbial tests and resistance profile. However, one should first try to eliminate the super infection by mechanical treatment and the use of Chlorhexidine gel. Renewed bacterial tests after this treatment would point the way forward in the follow-up treatment.

The presence of Fungi is a complicating factor in any infection. Fungi and bacteria are normally in balance, but super-infection by fungi is not uncommon following antibiotic treatment. Therefore, microbiological tests showing specific bacteria as well as fungi calls for the pre-treatment of the fungi. Sometimes, a combination of mechanical and Chlorhexidine treatment is sufficient. If specific antifungal therapy is needed, the choiceis: Nystatin 500 000 IU x 3 per day for 25 days.

We do not recommend Flukonazol because it is said to create resistance, and this should not be the dentist's choice to make.

The patients should be instructed to avoid sugar in their diets, since sugar is a potential fungal substrate, and to eat yoghurt or pharmaceutical products that adds lactic bacteria to the intestinal flora, which should be a biological way of suppressing the fungus.
After 4 weeks a new *bacterial* test will be helpful for selecting the antibacterial drug to take care of the bacteria involved.

Local antibiotic formulas

In order to be effective an antibiotic must reach its target area in adequate concentration, and stay there long enough to affect targeted bacteria. Target area, time and concentration are, therefore, important factors in deciding the effectiveness of the therapy.

Target area

The target area for antibiotic or chemotherapeutic treatment of periodontal disease is the periodontal pocket. Any compound, solid or liquid, which is brought into the oral cavity, does not penetrate into the periodontal pocket, even if kept in the mouth for a long time. In order to subject the periodontal pocket to any compound, there are two options: administer relatively large doses systemically, or to place the compound directly into the pocket.

Rinsing with water solutions of Chlorhexidine will have effect on the bacteria on the surfaces of the oral cavity *per se*, but have no or negligible effect on the sub-gingival bacterial flora. However, an important feature of Chlorhexidine is that it binds to various surfaces of the oral cavity, being released to the oral environment over a 12-hour period following application. Chlorhexidine may thus have a positive impact in the treatment of gingivitis or in the periods directly after surgery. Today, Chlorhexidine is used mainly as an effective plaque preventive compound for shorter periods, in patients who have problems performing efficient oral hygiene practices.

Concentration

To achieve an adequate result from an antibiotic, the antibiotic must reach the target area in a concentration that exceeds the concentration of target bacteria. On the other hand, we want to limit the concentration in order to eliminate the side effects. Thus, one has to be familiar with the MIC (Minimum Inhibitory Concentration) and MBC (Minimum Bactericidal Concentration) of the compound. These measures are assessed *In Vitro*. However, these measurements and their results cannot directly be applied to the situation in the periodontal pocket, in which several modifying factors may serve to reduce the efficacy of an antibiotic. In general, studies have indicated that the concentration might need increasing up to 50 times the MIC or MBC in order to achieve a desired clinical effect in the target area.
However, new systematic review shows little or neglible effect of these local drugs on periodontal disease.

Antibiotic drugs for local administration against periodontitis

Elyzol 25% dental gel (metronidazol) from ALPHARMA is approved for clinical use in the Scandinavian countries. Dentomycine (Minocycline) from American Cyanamide is already approved in Great Britain and Japan, whereas Acticite (a thread containing 0.52mg Minocycline/cm) from Meda/Alza corporation is approved in Sweden, Great Britain and Japan. Recently, Perio Products Ltd, Israel introduced Periochip (2.5mg Chlorhexidingluconate), and Atridox (19% Doxicyclin, Block Drug Co. Inc. USA). The advantage of these antibiotic chips, gels, fibers, etc. is that they may be introduced directly into the periodontal pocket, the target area. This means that it is possible to reduce the total dose, but maintain a very high concentration locally. This reduces the possibilities for some side effects.

The fact that these drugs have to be manually placed by a clinician, secures compliance. Another advantage of the local administration of drugs is that due to the enormous concentrations achieved, even bacteriostatic antibiotics such as Minocycline, become bactericidal. The disadvantage of local administration of the drugs is that target bacteria located in other areas are not reached. Also local administration of drugs, will not effect the microorganisms that have invaded the periodontal tissues. However, irrespective these limitations, local administration of drugs provides a small, though valuable addition to armamentarium for the treatment of periodontal diseases on an individualized basis, which is one of the most important concepts introduced in this book.

Elyzol 25% Dental Gel (ALPHARMA) is a metronidazole benzoate, which is mixed with a biodegradable compound. When the metronidazole benzoate is inserted into the temperate and moist pocket, it will flow into all parts of the pocket. The moisture will immediately start to cause separation of the active metronidazole from the benzoate. This happens over a period of 24 hrs, during which time the concentration of metronidazole greatly exceeds the MIC 50 values of all periodontal pathogens (except *A. actinomycetemcomitans*). The minute amounts of metronidazole found in serum is probably due to swallowing.

Acticite 0.52mg/cm (MEDA) are hollow fibers containing tetracycline. It is sold in lengths of 30cm, and is cut according to the need. The fibers are placed manually into the periodontal pocket following scaling and root planing, and all left there for 10 days. During this period, the tetracycline is released from the fibers, which gives a prolonged effect on the microbial flora in the target areas. The technique seems effective, but is very time consuming and operator sensitive. Fibers that are expelled from the pockets before 7 days should be replaced, but after 8 days, replacement is unnecessary. Since mechanical oral hygiene procedures easily may displace the fibers, the manufacturer suggests oral hygiene should be maintained though rinsing with Chlorhexidine. The manufacturer claims that the product provides 150x higher concentration in the target sites, and at the same time decreases the total dose by 98.9% as compared to systemic administration. Measurable tetracycline concentrations in the serum during this treatment have not been observed.

Atridox from Block Drug Corporation is a bioabsorbable gel made from poly-DL-lactide with 10% Doxicyline. *In vivo* studies have shown that MIC for most oral bacteria are sufficient for 7–8 days. Extensive clinical studies have shown reduced pocket depth of 2mm respectively.

Very few side effects have been reported, and few are expected as more experience is gained. Transitional tenderness at the site and local erythema are minor side effects. Allergies, though infrequent, are more serious possibilities. When tetracycline is diluted in water, the pH for the solution drops to 1–1.5. This has in some cases produced severe, but transitional, pulpal pains in the adjacent teeth. Abscess formation due to resistant microorganisms has also been reported.

Dentomycine is a semi-synthetic tetracycline (minocycline) in an ointment formulation. The product is made by American Cyanamide, and has proven effective in clinical studies. The product claims the same areas of indication and use as the other formulas mentioned above.

Resistance developments associated with the local formulations of Metronidazole and tetracycline have not been studied in depth. Only a few studies have been performed this area, and indicate that resistance development and the bactericidal effect is minimal due to the very high local dose in the periodontal pocket. However, some antibiotic will be discharged over the gingival margin in the course of the 1–10 days of placement and may lead to resistance development in the oral and intestinal flora. Other unwanted side effects over time are the increased incidence of fungal infections and occasional abscess formation by resistant bacteria.

Periochip (Proctor & Gamble) is a Chlorhexidingluconate (2.5mg) which is part of a biodegradable gelatin film. The gelatin film is placed manually into the pocket, where the active substance is discharged over a period of 10 days. *In vitro* studies show that 40% of the active substance is released, during the first 4 days, and the rest is released over the last 6 days.

The common side effect of Chlorhexidine such as staining of teeth, is not a problem in this formulation, since the amount of active substance that reaches the oral cavity is negligible. Some patients have reported only minute discomfort during the actual depositioning of the Periochip into the pocket.

All local antibiotic formulations are suggested used together with scaling and root planning. So far, studies have shown good result on the parameters of inflammation, but there is no indication that any of these formulations have a positive impact on the attachment level. The indication for use of the local antibiotics is the same as for the systemic formulation, and the strategy does not change. However, as shown through systematic reviews and meta analyses there is little to not detectable effect of the use of local antibiotics on periodontal disease.

The use of locally administered antibacterial agents is first and foremost the case of periodontal diseases that do not respond to adequate mechanical treatment, despite the fact that the patient has a flawless oral hygiene, and where microbiological tests show the presence of specific, periodontopathic microorganisms.

The patient should be informed not to use any mechanical oral hygiene measures the first day when applying Dentomycine, Elyzol 25% dental gel, and Atridox. When using Acticite, the manufacturer recommends refraining from mechanical oral hygiene for the full treatment of 10 days, and to maintain control of supragingival plaque by daily rinsing with Chlorhexidine.

For those who want to read more about antibiotic treatment of periodontal diseases we highly recommend:

Edwin Winkel Thesis. Systemic Antibiotic Therapy in Periodontics. 2000.

CHAPTER 5

Advanced Periodontal Surgical Techniques

Irrespective of treatment modality used, the primary goal is to arrest the progression of the disease and to cure the patient. Once this goal has been achieved, we can try to regenerate the lost periodontal tissues. The basic periodontal surgery as part of the treatment of periodontitis was discussed in Chapter 3. This chapter will briefly deal with different techniques for periodontal regeneration and mucogingival or periodontal plastic surgery.

It ought to be of interest for the general practitioner, and also for the dental hygienist, to be familiar with such advanced surgical procedures in order to be able to identify and refer suitable patients for such treatments in time for a successful treatment outcome.

It is important to know which type of defects are treatable, what can be expected as treatment outcome, how the treatment is performed, what follow-ups and supportive care are needed, and how achieved treatment results are maintained. This knowledge serves to provide optimal treatments for our patients.

Periodontal surgery with membranes

Regenerative periodontal surgery can be performed for the following periodontal defects:
1. Infrabony defects, primarily 2 and 3-wall defects

2. Class II furcation defects
3. Gingival recessions.

Periodontal wound healing

A periodontal defect surgically treated may heal spontaneously with some, but seldom with a complete regeneration of the defect, resulting in some probing depth reduction and partial regaining of clinical attachment. Follow-up radiographs can be very encouraging (Fig.21).
However, radiographic evidence of bone fill does not guarantee new attachment formation. During early healing downgrowth of the long junctional epithelium (and its in-

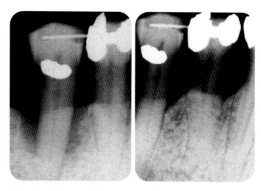

Fig 21 Pre- and postoperative roentgenograms showing bone fill following modified Widman flap procedure. (Note the immobilization of the mobile tooth 45 – fixing should be applied in cases where involved teeth are mobile)

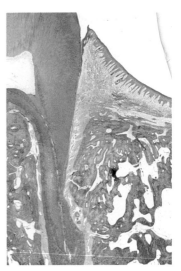

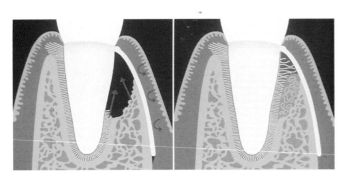

Fig 22 a Drawn images of the principles of GTR-treatment of infrabony periodontal defects. After surgically raising a flap and carefully scaled and root planed the defect a barrier is placed over the defect. The barrier is guiding the wound healing by primarily hampering the down growth of epithelial cells into the defect. (Courtesy of K. G. Edung)

Fig 22 b Histology of newly formed supporting tissue following the procedures described in Fig 22 a; Root cementum, periodontal fibres and alveolar bone. (Courtesy of K. G. Edung)

terposition between the root surface and the newly formed bone) may have prevented the formation of new attachment. True regeneration, and the formation of new cementum, new periodontal ligament and new supporting bone can only occur if epithelial cells are excluded from the healing area.

Guided tissue regeneration – GTR – is a surgical treatment modality that was developed during the early 1980s by Drs Thorkild Karring and Sture Nyman based on a series of studies on periodontal wound healing. They showed that periodontal regeneration is possible under certain conditions. The principle is based on preventing downgrowth of gingival connective tissue and epithelium by placing a surgical barrier membrane between the infrabony defect and the gingival flap before the flap is repositioned and sutured (Fig. 22 a). In the space thus created, a coagulum

is formed into which only cells from the surrounding bone and adjacent periodontal ligament can grow and theoretically form new attachment.

The purpose of the barrier membrane is to stabilize the blood clot and to allow only the desired cells to migrate towards the root surface and secure the formation of new cementum, insertion of new collagen fibers and the formation of new functional, alveolar bone by excluding non-desired cells. Animal as well as human histologies of GTR-treated infrabony and furcation defects have demonstrated the formation of new attachment, and several clinical studies have demonstrated that GTR-treatment of infrabony defects and of class II furcation defects is superior to other new attachment procedures in terms of obtaining clinical attachment gain and bone regeneration.

GTR – a technique sensitive treatment modality

Guided tissue regeneration is a treatment modality with a modest treatment outcome, provided the procedure is performed by a skilled operator, on the right defect, and in the right patient. Following elevation of mucoperiostal full thickness buccal and lingual flaps, the defect is carefully debrided, all granulation tissue is removed, the root surface is scaled and planed, and the barrier membrane is fitted firmly to the tooth. In order to accomplish periphery sealing and to prevent membrane collapse into the defect, the membrane must cover the defect and at least 3mm of the surrounding bone. The flaps are then mobilized, adjusted and sutured to completely cover the membrane.

Although the soft tissue management is basically the same as with a conventional MWF-procedure, it is extremely important that:
- The defect is properly debrided
- The bony walls are decorticated to facilitate bleeding into the defect
- The flaps are sutured to complete interproximal closure and membrane coverage without flap tension.

The decortication is made in order to obtain enough fresh blood for the formation of a coagulum within which vessels and cells can form and create new attached tissues. The membrane tends to stabilize the blood clot. However, the placement of a barrier membrane between the flaps and the underlying bone may compromise the blood supply to the flaps. This might make healing more difficult, resulting in flap necrosis and retraction. Such dire development can be prevented by:
1. Making an incision that goes deep interproximally in order to preserve the original papillae or elongating the papillae by scalloping the buccal flap. The papillae should be kept as thick as possible, but attached granulation tissue must be removed.
2. Releasing incision. Before repositioning the buccal flap, a horizontal releasing incision is made at the base of the flap, and a sharp dissection above the periosteum is made in apical direction. This will significantly increase the mobility of the flap and enable the suturing of the flap in a more coronal position. If the flap is initially scalloped buccally, this will result in increased root exposure, but the increased mobility of the flap will accomplish the root to be covered.
3. Tension free suturing. The papillae are joined interproximally with a (modified) mattress suture, which actually are sutures traditionally used to line the button holes in Norwegian, male traditional folk-suites.

Notice that the sutures keep the flaps in a coronal position. Surgical dressing should not be used. If non-resorbable barrier membranes are used they are removed after 4–6 weeks. Post-surgical exposure of the membrane can make earlier removal necessary.

Post-surgical instruction and care

The post-surgical instructions and follow-up are very similar to those following any periodontal surgery with a few exceptions:
1. The sutures should be kept in place as long as they hold, preferably for 3–4 weeks
2. Rinsing with Chlorhexidine solution is extended to 6–8 weeks. During the last 3–4 weeks, rinsing can be exchanged with local application of Chlorhexidine gel applied with an impression syringe
3. Mechanical tooth cleaning is not resumed until 6–8 weeks or 1 week after a non-resorbable membrane has been removed.

Prognosis for GTR therapy

The prognosis for GTR therapy is dependent on the defect morphology, how deep the defect is in relation to the amount of remaining periodontal ligament, and the availability of progenitor cells that can repopulate the wound. Other factors of importance to optimize the outcome are the operator's knowledge and skill, as well as patient compliance. Patient collaboration in the post-surgical care program is paramount. Smoking may compromise the soft tissue healing over the membrane, which may lead to early membrane exposure.

The expectations of new attachment following GTR therapy should be realistic. Not all periodontal tissues lost through the disease might be expected to be restored. This has been borne out in several clinical studies. However, even a few mm of attachment gain can prove crucial for the prognosis of the tooth, and determine the entire treatment strategy. For example, an initial 10mm deep infrabony defect at the mesial aspect of a maxillary canine can at the one-year re-examination show a clinical attachment level gain of 7mm and a bone fill of 5mm as evaluated radiographically. In a recent study, a compilation of data from a large number of clinical studies on GTR treatment of intrabony defects showed that with intrabony defects $\geq$ 4mm, clinical attachment gain averaged 70%, with a bone fill averaging 50% of the defect depth.

It is important not only to evaluate the outcome of GTR therapy radiographically, but to consider pocket depth reduction and the gain of clinical attachment as the primary treatment outcome variables.

In recent systematic reviews membrane therapy only showed limited value in treating defects following periodontal disease.

Membrane products

There are quite a number of GTR barrier products available on the international market, ranging from very simple Teflon membranes to more complicated synthetic materials. Basically, membranes are either resorbable or non-resorbable. The resorbable membranes have the advantage over the non-resorbable in that a second surgery for their removal is unnecessary. The following is a description of some of the marketed membranes:

1. **Gore-tex periodontal material** (W.L. Gore & Associates, Flagstaff, Arizona, USA) was the first commercially available barrier specifically designed for periodontal regeneration. It was made of expanded Ply-Tetra-Fluoro-Ethylene (ePTFE). This membrane barrier was used in the majority of clinical studies. A further development of this membrane is the Gore-tex TR (Titanium Re-enforced). This re-inforced membrane is able to prevent the membrane from falling into the defect, and thereby secure the space needed for regeneration to occur.
2. **Resolut** (W.L. Gore). This is a resorbable membrane based on a co-polymer composition polyglycolide/polylactide with a polyglycolide fiber net on the surface to accomplish integration. It is probably the most used resorbable membrane on the market, although collagen based membranes are increasing their share on the market. It is a somewhat stiff and difficult to work with, and may need extra training. Fairly good clinical results have been reported, although somewhat inferior to those using the regular Gore-tex non-resorbable membranes.
3. **Bio Gide** (Geistlich AG Switzerland). This a collagen membrane of bovine origin. The material is slowly resorbed and barrier function is claimed to be main-

tained for 4–6 months. The resorption is through proteolysis. This is a very interesting product that was originally developed for bone augmentation and implants in conjunction with Bio-os, a bovine bone substitute.

4. **Vicryl Periodontal Mesh** (Johnson & Johnson, USA). This is the pioneer membrane from a company, well known from the production of resorbable suture material. The membrane material is a co-polymer polyglycolide/polylactide.9:1. The material resorbs by hydrolysis, which is probably too fast to offer any broader usage.

Periodontal regeneration with Enamel Matrix Proteins – Emdogain

A different biological concept for periodontal regeneration is Emdogain (Biora, Lund, Sweden). Emdogain is an enamel matrix protein consisting of amelogenins developed from pig jaw tooth germs. The development of this product stems from research by Professor Lars Hammarstrom et al. at the Karolinska Institute, Huddinge, Sweden, and the knowledge on embryological tooth development and the role of amelogenins in the development of root cementum. The concept is, that Emdogain when applied to the cleaned and dry root surface will allow mesenchymal cells in the blood clot to develop into cementoblasts. Animal and human histology studies have demonstrated that properly performed, the treatment will result in the formation of new cementum, periodontal ligament and bone. Clinical data are currently being presented, and tend to show gain of clinical attachment and bone as well as pocket reduction of clinical significance.

One of the clinical advantages with Emdogain is that it can be used in several defects at the same time, Following incision, elevation of flaps with careful preservation of the papillae, debridement of the defect etc., scaling and root planing, the root surface is 'conditioned' for 3 minutes with 24% EDTA gel to demineralize the root surface and remove smear layers. The area is then profusely irrigated with saline, the root surface is dried and the Emdogain gel is applied with a syringe to fill the entire defect with some excess. The carrier substance is rapidly absorbed during the initial healing, leaving the active components on the root surface.

In recent systematic reviews Emdogain only shows limited value in the treatment of periodontal infrabony defects.

Economical aspects

Regenerative periodontal surgery may sometimes offer a good alternative to tooth extraction and more expensive prosthodontic treatment. Also, maintaining ones own teeth is to many people a matter of life quality. Regenerative treatment has also been shown to be successful in the treatment of severely compromised bridge abutments.

In times when restorative dental treatment becomes gradually more expensive, it is important for everyone involved in dental care to provide the best treatment to the least cost. Knowing the periodontal defects in which regenerative treatment will be predictably successful, is therefore important.

Important questions to raise in choosing between various regenerative methods:
1. Is the suggested treatment modality well documented from well-designed clinical studies published in peer reviewed journals?
2. If so, has the method shown itself to be significantly effective, and are there methods evaluated in well-designed studies

that show clinically relevant results in comparison with others?

3. Is the operator who intends to do the procedure experienced with the technique and can show good results?

4. How good is the prognosis for the suggested treatment? Alternatively how necessary is the suggested treatment for the longevity of the tooth?

Periodontal plastic surgery (muco-gingival surgery)

Periodontal plastic surgery (PPS) is gradually becoming more and more important as part of esthetic dentistry. PPS includes:

1. Treatment of gingival recession defects on various indications and etiology
2. Treatment of unfavorably attached frenulae, primarily in the mandibular anterior area and lack of or inadequate amounts of keratinized/attached gingiva
3. Surgical crown-lengthening to improve soft tissue esthetics, mainly in the maxillary anterior areas, but also as pre-prosthetic surgery for improving gingival architecture and esthetics, and to create optimal retention in endodontically treated teeth that will be used as abutments, or teeth with severe loss of substance
4. Soft tissue augmentation in areas with big concavities due to loss of underlying bone caused by e.g. traumatic tooth extraction.

In this chapter only a few methods for the treatment of gingival recessions will be briefly discussed.

Miller's classification
The US periodontist P.D. Miller defines gingival recessions according to 4 classes and the Miller classifications are used for determining possible treatment outcomes.

Class 1 (Fig. 23 a) Gingival recession that does not extend to the muco-gingival border. No loss of interproximal soft or hard tissue. 100% root coverage should be expected.

Class II (Fig. 23 a) Gingival recession that extends to or beyond the muco-gingival border. No loss of interproximal soft or hard tissue. 100% root coverage should be expected.

Class III (Fig. 23 c) Gingival recession that does not extend to the muco-gingival border. Loss of interproximal soft or hard tissue and /or displaced tooth mesially or distally that will prevent 100% root coverage. Partial root coverage should be expected.

Class IV (Fig. 23 d) Gingival recession that extends to or beyond the muco-gingival border. Loss of interproximal soft or hard tissue and /or displaced tooth mesially or distally that will prevent 100% root coverage. Partial root coverage should be expected.

Gingival recessions are usually in areas with a narrow alveolar process and lack of marginal buccal bone. Superimposed on this anatomical problem is trauma from over-excessive tooth brushing, tongue- or lip piercing, (Fig. 24) ornaments, orthodontic treatment, parafunction, etc. It should be stressed that we are not talking about periodontitis related defects. However, if in addition to the gingival recession there is periodontitis, the prognosis may be less favorable.

There are several treatment modalities for gingival recessions. However, as with periodontitis the cause of the lesions – usually over-excessive or incorrect tooth brushing – should be dealt with. Prior to the corrective surgery, the patient needs to learn to perform a careful roll stroke brushing technique and to use extra-soft brushes.

In case of piercing this should be removed. Fig. 24 shows excessive gingival destruction lingual in lower jaw due to tongue piercing.

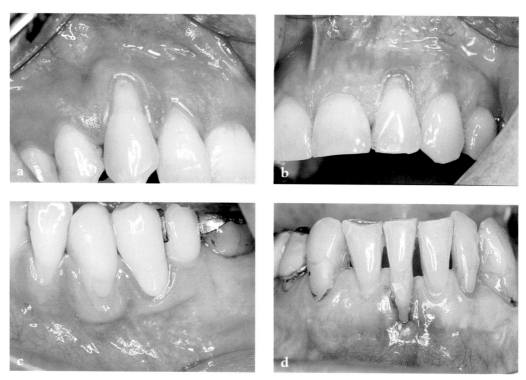

Fig 23 a – d Example of gingival retractions according to Miller's classification; a) Class I, b) Class II, c) Class III, d) Class IV.

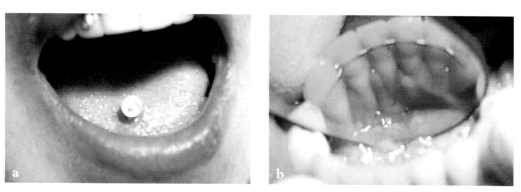

Fig 24 a,b Piercing of tongue and ornament which has caused considerable gingival destruction lingual on 43, 42 and 41 in a 22 year-old woman.

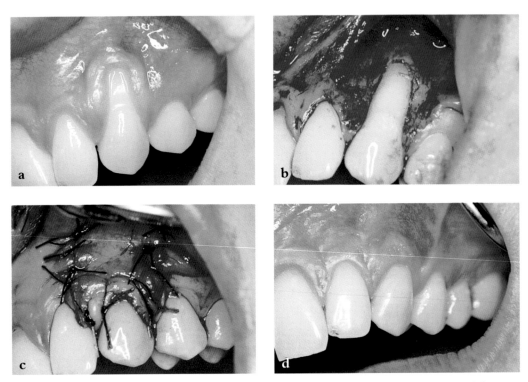

Fig 25 a – d Treatment of a gingival retraction 23 (Miller Class I) by coronally repositioned flap surgery. a) The exposed root surface thoroughly cleaned, b) Trapezoid flap raised exposing a healthy root surface not covered by bone. c) The flap is repositioned coronally and sutured without tension to the remaining attached gingival/mucus membrane on each side. d) a stable clinical image 18 months after surgery.

Coronally repositioned flaps

This is the most commonly used and easiest method for the treatment of Miller Class I and II defects (Fig. 25 a). A prerequisite for this technique is that there is some with keratinized gingiva left. The procedure can involve one or several teeth simultaneously. Before the incision the exposed root surface is properly scaled and planed – unless there is calculus or a caries lesion polishing with pumice and rubber cup is sufficient – to the bottom of the gingival sulcus. The root surface may also be conditioned with saturated citric acid or EDTA-gel. The area is irrigated with water. Two apically diverging incisions are made, starting at the level of half the recession going into bone and extended all the way down to the level of the vestibule. A full thickness flap is raised to a level just apical of the buccal bone crest. Often the root is exposed beyond the gingival recession. If there is no periodontal pathology present, this exposed surface of the root is covered with healthy periodontal ligament and cementum, and should be left untouched or at least not instrumented. A horizontal incision is next made through the periosteum, and a partial thickness flap is dissected sharply with the scalpel just above the periosteum. Provided all collagen fibers of the flap and the periosteum are severed, the flap is sufficiently modified to be coronally advanced without tension. Notice that every remaining periostal fiber will offer resistance to the mobility of the flap and therefore has to be severed. The remaining part of the papillae is now de-epithelialized (Fig. 25 b) to create a wound bed to which the coronally advanced flap is sutured. The first suture is a sling suture 4-0 through the flap papillae, around the neck of the tooth to keep the flap in position and against the de-epithelialized papillae. The vertical incisions are preferably sutured with 5-0 fast resorbable Vicryl or catgut sutures (Fig. 25 c). No periodontal pack should be used, but a light curing dressing could be applied to protect the wound during the initial healing. Post-surgical problems are rare, but some edema can occur since the periosteum has been elevated.

Post-surgical instructions and follow-up is the same as with any other periodontal surgery:

- Inform the patient that some swelling may occur
- No mechanical tooth cleaning in the area for 2–3 weeks.
- Mouth rinsing with Chlorhexidine solution 0.2% 2–3 times daily
- Soft food intake for 2 weeks (pasta, soups, patè etc.)
- Call your dentist if discomfort arises.

Sutures are removed after 7–10 days. Careful tooth brushing with roll strokes can be resumed after 2–3 weeks. Fig. 25 d shows a stable situation 18 months after the surgery.

Coronally repositioned flap with subepithelial connective tissue graft

This method is based on the principle of the coronally advanced flap procedure, and is used when keratinized tissue is lacking and/or when the tissue is extremely thin. It is a technically more demanding procedure, and post-surgical pain from the donor area is quite frequent. Preparation of the recipient bed is performed in a manner similar to that of the normal coronally advanced flap procedure, with the exception that it is usually only a split thickness flap. The palatal donor area is prepared; a horizontal incision is made palatally at the area of the first premolar to the first molar; and a subepithelial connective tissue graft of sufficient size is dissected free. The graft is tested and trimmed to fit the recipient wound and sutured. The flap is then coronally advanced to cover a major part but not necessarily all of the graft. The exposed part of the graft will survive and heal, and will in due time be covered with keratinized epithelium. Also the palatal wound is sutured with a 5-0 suture. Both wounds may be covered with light curing dressing. Post-surgical care and follow-up as normal.

Both these treatment modalities have shown very good results and good coverage, when properly performed on the correct indications. Biologically the mode of healing against the tooth is through a long junctional epithelium, perhaps with some connective tissue adhesion.

As an alternative to the subepithelial connective tissue graft GTR has been suggested. A membrane should both contribute to healing with the formation of new attachment and increased thickness of the soft tissue. For this a space has to be created and maintained between the membrane and the root surface. Today there are no ideal resorbable membranes fulfilling these demands. The Gore-tex TR ePTFE mem-

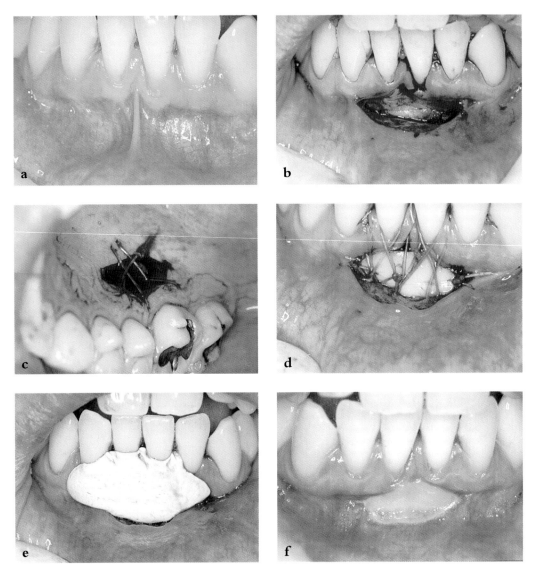

Fig 26 a – f Enhancing the surface of attached gingiva by an epithelialized connective tissue graft.

branes are very suitable, but necessitate two surgical sessions within 6 weeks. Therefore, they will never constitute a real alternative to the connective tissue graft.

Epithelialized connective tissue graft – 'free gingival graft'

The free gingival graft procedure is mainly used to increase the width of attached gingiva in the mandibular anterior region, where gingival recession has occurred due to frenulum pull (Fig. 26). Very often two or more adjacent teeth are involved. For the treatment of single recessions a free gingival graft is esthetically less than satisfactory. The grafted tissue usually becomes too thick, and more often than not, the color of the graft does not match.

An incision is made in the mucogingival border along the entire defect, and is terminated with a slightly oblique releasing incision. A split flap is then dissected by sharp supraperiostal incision. The wound edge is apically displaced and sutured to the periosteum (Fig.

26 b). In the palate an area of the same size as the recipient site is prepared. The graft is dissected free, transferred to the recipient bed, checked, reshaped and sutured with the use of resorbable catgut sutures (Fig. 26 d). The graft is immobilized with Coe-Pac (Fig. 26 e) or light curing dressing. Also the donor wound is sutured and covered.

The post-surgical care is the same as following any PPS procedure, including twice daily rinsing with a 0.2% Chlorhexidine solution until tooth brushing can be resumed. Some temporary discomfort and swelling in the cheek and some pain in the donor wound can be expected during the first week. The dressing and non-resorbed suture remnants are removed after 7–10 days (Fig. 26 f).

Apart from these quite easy to do PPS procedures there are the sliding flap, the double papilla flap and the envelope technique with or without subepithelial connective tissue graft. These procedure are generally more difficult to perform, and should therefore in general be performed by experienced periodontists.

CHAPTER 6

Follow-up and Maintenance

The follow-up and maintenance phase is every bit as important as a complete diagnosis and an effective treatment of periodontal diseases. The first reexamination should be performed 3–6 months after the active treatment was completed. It is really not important to recall a patient earlier, unless inadequate collaboration regarding oral hygiene is expected, or the presence of a specific infection is anticipated. A recall program should ensure the control of the individual patient's needs. Too frequent recalls may lead to over treatment and patient fatigue. It is prudent to remember that healing following periodontal therapy implies resolution of the entire inflammatory immunopathological circumstance, and that the body must have time to react to the treatment and the repair. Hygiene controls may of course be performed more frequently, but should not be warranted unless the patient's performance was dubious in the past. Good oral hygiene should be a normal part of a periodontal patient's daily routine, and it is of the essence that the dentist or hygienist approaches the hygiene controls seriously, and never lowers the standards that the clinician and the patient agreed upon. *If hygiene standards are lowered, the treatment will fail.*

The first post-treatment evaluation should contain assessments of:
• The patient's cooperation

• The gingival response to treatment
• The treatment strategy evaluation.

What one may expect is:
• Low plaque scores (<20% surfaces with plaque).
• Elimination or reduction in gingival inflammation (few surfaces with bleeding)
• A markedly reduced number of surfaces with pocket depth > 4mm

Pockets with a reduced measurable depth of ending of 4–5mm should also be assessed in terms of tissue firmness and tone. Such pockets with no bleeding may be regarded as 'symptoms' of earlier disease. But at the same time these 'scars' are sites we may have to accept 'as is'. They represent sites where disease may recur, and should thus be kept under continuous observation. The periodontal attachment level is the most precise, measurable representation of success or failure. Signs of continuing loss of attachment is a clear indication of the need for new or continuing treatment (see treatment strategies Chapter 7).

Roentgenological control is indicated approximately one year after treatment. This is the time it takes for X-rays to reveal both quantitative changes in bone level (filling of bone defects, continuous bone loss), and qualitative changes (like bone density and the density of the *lamina durae*). While in-

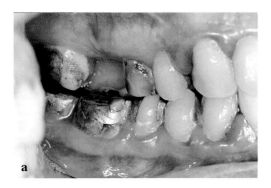

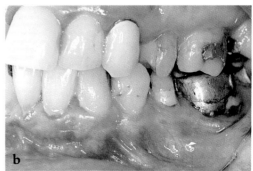

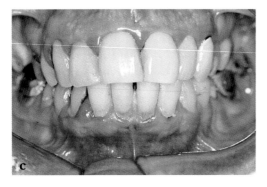

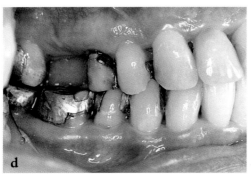

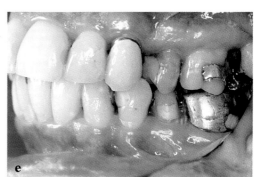

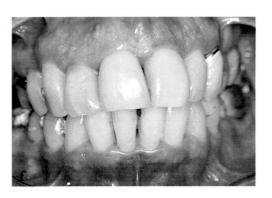

Fig 27 a – f An example of the effect of a thoroughly and adequately performed non-surgical periodontal treatment in a patient with flawless oral hygiene. The gingival inflammation is gone, gingiva is retracted, tough and firm. All pockets have been eliminated.

creased density and/or amount of bone are good signs, a reduced level and reduced density are signs of continuing disease.

If the result of treatment is satisfactory, a maintenance program is designed to suit the individual patient. If the result is unsatisfactory, the reasons for this may be sought among the various important variables described in the previous chapters of this book: insufficient oral hygiene, insufficient treatment, specific infections, reinfection, or other reasons such as stress, immunological problems, systemic diseases, etc. (see treatment strategies Chapter 7).

Supportive treatment

The goals of supportive treatment are:
- Increasing the general health condition of the patient
- Reduction of the risk for recurrence of disease, and
- Preventing the recurrence of disease, and the development of new disease.

Several long-term studies have shown that adequate supportive treatment is necessary to prevent recurrence and development of new disease in all patients that have been treated for periodontal diseases. The main problem is to decide how often such controls should be carried out. This decision depends on the risk for recurrence of or new disease in the individual patient including:
- The type and severity of the disease
- The general health of the patient
- The age of the patient in relation to type and severity of the infection, and
- The presence of risk factors at the individual, as well as on tooth level.

Risk factors at the individual level

- Collaboration >30% FMP (Full Mouth Plaque score)

- The number of sites with BOP (Bleeding on Probing)>25%
- A high number of (> 6) residual pockets >5mm
- General disease (i.e. Diabetes mellitus, rheumatic disease, depressions etc.)
- Smoking > 10 cigarettes per day.

Tooth level

- Furcation involvements
- Residual periodontal tissue support less than 1/3 of the length of the root
- Increased, or increasing mobility.

Site Level

- Repeated bleeding on probing (BOP)
- Residual probing pocket depth > 5mm
- Increasing pocket depth > 2mm.

Example: For a patient in his 30s who has been treated for advanced periodontitis (aggressive) the supportive treatment should be conducted every third month. A patient in his 50s that has experienced general bone loss including more than 1/3 of the length of the root, in combination with residual pockets of 4–5mm, probably does not require more frequent follow-ups than once or twice a year.

Apart from oral hygiene control and reinstruction regarding risk teeth and sites, subgingival cleaning should be concentrated on risk teeth and areas, or teeth and surfaces that display clear signs of progression.

Summary

Successful treatment of periodontal diseases implies adequate and regular maintenance care in order to achieve continuous periodontal health. Following active treatment, regardless of strategy applied, a maintenance program based on the individual patient and the presence of risk factors, should be instituted.

The clinician is responsible for the maintenance care, which must include the patient's general health, plaque control, periodontal diagnosis; and when needed, subgingival scaling and root planing. At the first sign of recurring disease, consideration must be given to an assessment of microbiological and immunological factors and antibiotic therapy.

CHAPTER 7

Strategies when treating periodontal diseases. A summary

We have continuously asked ourselves why such a widespread and often devastating disease as periodontitis receives so little attention in the dental office. We believe that the reason is that the patient often experiences continuing bone loss – even after treatment and flawless oral hygiene. It even happens that patients lose bone despite treatment by specialists in periodontics. There is a widespread feeling among general practitioners that known treatment of periodontitis does not help, so "why treat anyway?"

If we want a better collective quality of the diagnosis and treatment of periodontal diseases, we need to change the clinicians' perception of what periodontal disease actually is, and that it is possible to treat these diseases adequately. We need to convey to the clinician that every periodontitis patient is different and needs individual treatment. Last but not least, clinicians should recognize that there is a need for a stringent diagnosis and treatment strategy. If one wants to work with periodontal diseases seriously, one must adapt from being a dentist to becoming a specialist in infection medicine.

In this chapter we try to summarize how, with the aid of the content of the 6 foregoing chapters, it is possible to diagnose and design various treatment strategies for different periodontal diseases. It is not of much help to give general recommendations, since the individual therapist must gain experience with this part of infection medicine while working on it. One of the most important realizations is that one recognizes the fact that there are several different periodontal diseases with complex levels of difficulty, and that many of them are so complex that they should be referred to the periodontist. Our first advice is: **contact a periodontist and start a collaboration.** If you do not wish to involve yourself in periodontal work, it is still important that you arrange that your patients receive optimal and adequate treatment. It is not embarrassing to refer a patient to a specialist – the embarrassing moment occurs when the patient realizes that he would have saved his teeth and a substantial amount of money, had you referred him to a specialist earlier on.

As elaborated on in chapter one, all periodontal diseases are different. Thus, the road to success in treating these infections starts with your intellectual acceptance of the fact that this is true, and that you intend to search for evidence confirming this. Then, start applying the strategies stringently, and thereby experience the success that comes with the correct selection of treatment. The main problem is that science has not yet recognized the entire clinical concept as presented in this treatise, although all parts are available. Therefore, it is necessary to test the power of the concept through personal work experiences.

The first step is to establish a very broad diagnosis of the case, and then to narrow it down to the actual periodontal infections. The clinical work takes more time than you are used to from working with previous clinical concepts. It is very important to keep in mind that the patient in fact suffers from the negative consequences of an adequate immunological reaction to a microbiological challenge. However, on the bright side, it is very convenient to have a patient under treatment for a long period since the hygiene routines are more easily developed when controlled and reinforced over a longer period. What you are used to through your previous work is that the patient has a good oral hygiene as long as he is under treatment, but that its quality is reduced over the weeks and months to come until the next visit. **The patient has not had the time and possibility to *incorporate* the hygiene routines into his daily routines.** Also, it is impossible to apply the rules behind the strategies when the intervals between the appointments are too short. A precise periodontal diagnosis may only be arrived at over time, and only after an initial mechanical treatment phase. The questions to ask are: Is this chronic periodontitis? Is it a specific infection, an immunological aberration, or all of the above?

Pre-treatment initial diagnosis

The first appointment must give the patient a sense of receiving something substantive while we 'speak' to them. The patient must feel that you are making progress, otherwise he will get suspicious, restless and disappointed that nothing happens. Such a situation will not serve to open the communication channels between the two of you. At this point, and in your own mind, this patient suffers from chronic periodontits and that's all that matters. Microbiologically, we initially regard all cases as non-specific infections (with very few exceptions). If the patient has a deficient oral hygiene, the pocket measurements may not be all that important since subsequent to improvement in oral hygiene, gingivitis levels will be reduced, edematous tissue will shrink, and pocket depth will be reduced. The patient must be thoroughly informed about the nature of periodontal diseases. This is extremely important, since this is a disease, which clearly needs the patient's cooperation in order for the treatment to be successful. Also, it is important to inform the patient of why you will do what, and why it might take some time do reach the goals. If these messages do not get through here, the treatment will fail. That is why the information, should be staged and limited during the first session. The important introductory message is: **"You suffer from a combination of infections, and we must sort out which infection is harmful, and which is reversible without damage."** Then, the patient should be taught how to perform an adequate oral hygiene, including the use of interdental brushes. The brush should be large enough that the surfaces of the approximal area are cleaned, but not so big as to cause damage to the tooth. The diameter of the brush most probably will have to be increased as the treatment proceeds and the gingival edema is reduced. INFORMED COLLABORATION is of the essence. Without it the treatment will fail. Another point, whatever oral hygiene procedure assign to the patient's oral home care, the routine will be broken if the patient is not able to buy the recommended products. So, hard-to-get oral hygiene equipment is no good, even if technically superior. Instead, settle for the second best, but which is readily accessible to the patient.

The next step is to let the patient get some time to himself to try out and personalize the procedures. If the patient has been informed, motivated and instructed in a language and manner that are understandable, it is rare to find one who will not perform as well as he possibly can, which normally is enough for long lasting success. It is important that the patient realizes the serous situation, and accepts responsibility over his own health. If the patient is informed, and still does not respond satisfactorily, a note to that effect should be made in the patient's record. This does not make the patient a lesser person, only one who has other priorities. This situation is extremely important to recognize; there is no use in an elaborate periodontal treatment, if the patient does not adequately perform the prescribed oral home care program. This must be conveyed to the patient. Every normally equipped person is responsible for himself. If the person suffers from reduced mental resources, his health is your responsibility and you must try your best to reach the patient. The communication should always be individualized. Remember that every person has his/her own periodontal disease, and every treatment is individualized. Communication is an important part of the treatment, and should be individualized as well. **The correct approach produces results – if the patient wants it.** When the hygiene is improving, it is important to demonstrate to patients that pocket depth has been reduced and that the disease has decreased in severity. The patient's homework has paid off. What better motivation can there be?

Subgingival scaling – treatment and diagnostics

The next step is to start the actual treatment. Scaling and root planing aim at the removal of supra- and subgingival plaque and calculus. This must also be individualized, through the choice of instruments, how you position yourself (and the patient) in relation to the patient and his anatomy and physiology. The instruments must be newly sharpened so you can effectively remove the pathological material. You must have a number of instrument cassettes, and a few special scalers needed in specific situations. The selection of instrument manufacturer is not important, as long as you like to hold the instruments and that they help you get the job done.

Subgingival scaling is time consuming. Also, the effectiveness of removal of sub-gingival calculus decreases with the increasing depth of the pockets. At some point surgery is necessary.

Optimal scaling and root planing is a non-specific treatment of a non-specific infection *as well as* a diagnostic tool for distinguishing between specific and non-specific infections in different diseases. The purpose is to reduce the amount of bacteria present in the target areas. If this does not help, and the patient's oral home care is unquestionable, this may be a sign that something else is at work. If you see the patient every third month from now on, he/she will either experience continuing good periodontal health, or continuing (or renewed) destruction in selected areas or in the entire dentition. If the lasting result is good, you have treated a non-specific infection and the long-term result is now dependent upon continued good oral hygiene practices. If destruction continues in selected or all areas treated, it is likely that this patient suffers from a specific infection, which does not naturally respond to the non-specific treatment.

The 'treatment resistant' – recalcitrant – refractory – periodontal disease

A lot of names for an inadequately treated periodontal disease. The pockets that did not respond to mechanical treatment should now be studied again. Was the scaling and root planing adequate? Were the instruments sharp enough? Were the interpretations of the clinical and roentgenological features correct? These questions can be answered in the affirmative, and the most common reason for failure is insufficient scaling and/or insufficient oral hygiene. If not, the possibility exists that the patient has a specific infection, and that microbiological tests are in order. At this point it is necessary to broaden the diagnostic arsenal and individualization of the diagnosis and the possibility for treatment.

Adjunct antibiotic treatment in periodontal disease control

A microbiological test is likely to disclose the presence and domination of specific pathogens. It is now time to decide which antibiotic/antibacterial drug to apply in eliminating these pathogens. When selecting an antibiotic, it must have clinically proven effect against the microorganisms described in the test. This may sound obvious, but an antimicrobial effect in the laboratory does not necessarily show the same efficacy within the periodontal pocket, where several factors will *counteract any substance introduced to* alter the microbiological balance. A large biomasse might reduce the effect of any antimicrobial substance, and the presence of microorganisms or substances that are able to bind, destroy or alter the antibiotic may also modify the effect of treatment. The knowledge of pocket ecology is as important as the resistance of the individual pathogens.

Incorrect choice of antibiotics may elicit serious side effects as well as influencing the general ecology. Therefore, we cannot emphasize enough how important the microbiological tests actually are. **Antibiotics used against periodontal diseases, without a proper microbiological test, is absolutely wrong.**

The selection of the most effective antibiotic based on a microbiological tests must be made according to a specific set of rules

1. *Antibiotic therapy in the treatment of periodontal diseases is not effective unless performed as an adjunct to repeated scaling and root planing.*

2. *Antibiotic therapy is not effective in the long term in patients with inadequate oral hygiene. Thus giving an antibiotic to patient with bad oral hygiene is wrong. In order to perform a microbiological test the patient must have exhibited good oral hygiene practices; and the dentist must have carried out an adequate scaling and root planing.*

3. *The selection criteria for the use of antibiotics based on different microbiological test results are described in Chapter 4.*

4. *As you see, the use of antibiotics in periodontal disease control is associated with a great deal of responsibility. The manufacturers of such products claim that the most common problems are reduced or eliminaed by using local antibiotics. However, they do not tell you about the inherent problems of using these products.*

The follow-up phase

The follow-up phase is of imperative importance. Hygiene controls with reinstruction and remotivation may be warranted if the self-care is dwindling. However, this is infrequently needed in those patients that have been given the appropriate time to develop a routine for this work (Chapter 2).

Routine controls should include checking of the oral hygiene practices, attachment level measurements and an update on the patients' general health. Today patients are frequently given new medications by their physicians, and it is important to keep track of their impact on the periodontal tissue. If antibiotic therapy was part of the actual periodontal treatment, a microbiological test may be made in order to evaluate the therapy. A combination of clinical, microbiological and general evaluation gives you the best position to say – "it's OK," or "there is something developing here, and we have to deal with it."

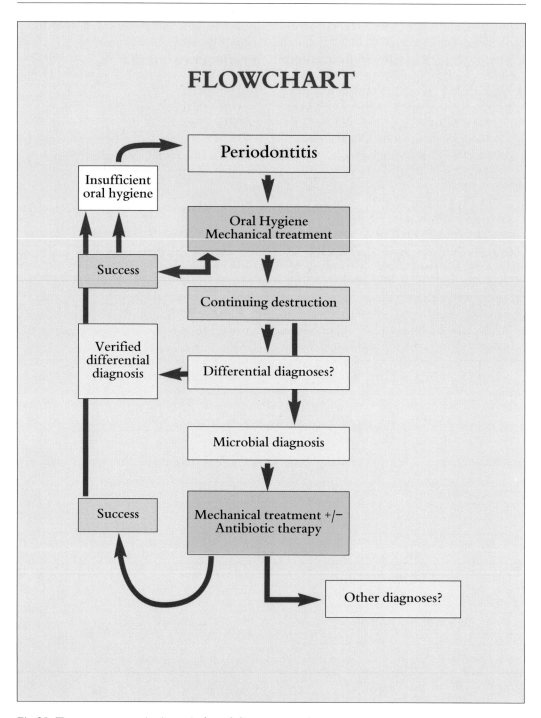

Fig 28 Treatment strategies in periodontal disease control.

Strategies for treatment of periodontal diseases

Establish a regular and close collaboration with a Periodontist, and refer the patient early so that the disease may not develop too far before being treated adequately.

Meticulous mechanical treatment (scaling and root planing) with or without surgical techniques constitutes the primary treatment of the periodontal disease. A post-treatment period of 3–6 months will reveal if the primary treatment has been a success or not.

If conventional mechanical treatment has failed; analyze all possible reasons for failure (inadequate treatment, or deficient oral hygiene, differential diagnosis).

If specific infection is suspected, perform microbiological tests.

If an antibiotic therapy is contemplated, select the correct antibiotic for the specific target bacteria based on your knowledge of the patient.

Antibiotics should be prescribed following repeated scaling and root planing, and for patients who, despite good oral hygiene, have shown a recurrence of disease.

The microbiological situation should be evaluated 3–12 months following the antibiotic treatment.